AIDS, DRUGS AND
SEXUAL RISK

AIDS, DRUGS AND SEXUAL RISK

LIVES IN THE BALANCE

Neil McKeganey and
Marina Barnard

OPEN UNIVERSITY PRESS
Buckingham · Philadelphia

Open University Press
Celtic Court
22 Ballmoor
Buckingham
MK18 1XW

and

1900 Frost Road, Suite 101
Bristol, PA 19007, USA

First Published 1992
Reprinted 1993

Library of Congress Cataloging-in-Publication Data
McKeganey, Neil P.
  AIDS, drugs, and sexual risk : lives in the balance / Neil
McKeganey and Marina Barnard.
    p.   cm.
  Includes bibliographical references and indexes.
  ISBN 0-335-09970-X (pbk.)   ISBN 0-335-09971-8 (hardback)
  1. AIDS (Disease)—Epidemiology.   2. AIDS (Disease)—Social
aspects.   3. Intravenous drug abuse.   I. Barnard, Marina, 1960–
II. Title.
  [DNLM: 1. HIV Infections—epidemiology.   2. Needle Sharing.
3. Risk Factors.   4. Sex Behavior.   5. Substance Abuse, Intravenous.
WD 308 M4778a]
RA644.A25M4   1992
614.5′993—dc20
DNLM/DLC
  for Library of Congress   91–46380
                                                                  CIP

Typeset by Inforum Typesetting, Portsmouth
Printed and bound in Great Britain by
Biddles Ltd, Guildford and King's Lynn

Dedication

To Michael Bloor, a sociologists' sociologist
and a friend

A mean wind wanders through the backcourt trash.
Hackles on puddles rise, old mattresses
puff briefly and subside. Play-fortresses
of brick and bric-a-brac spill out some ash.
Four storeys have no windows left to smash,
but in the fifth a chipped sill buttresses
mother and daughter the last mistresses
of that black block condemned to stand, not crash.
Around them the cracks deepen, the rats crawl.
The kettle whimpers on a crazy hob.
Roses of mould grow from ceiling to wall.
The man lies late since he has lost his job,
smokes on one elbow, letting his coughs fall
thinly into an air too poor to rob.

From *The Glasgow Sonnets* by Edwin Morgan (1982)

Contents

Foreword

The tragedy of HIV infection and AIDS has raised a number of issues about our society which are new, urgent, and previously neglected. Many of these concern hidden areas of life about which we previously knew little, and which are very difficult to research – drug use, prostitution, the sexual behaviour of those, especially young people, who may be most at risk. The study of these topics presents a considerable challenge.

The work described in this book was conducted as part of a programme of studies on behavioural aspects of HIV/AIDS funded by the Economic and Social Research Council. The aim of this programme, within the wider medical and social research initiative, has been to provide knowledge from which effective policies can be developed to combat the epidemic.

McKeganey and Barnard's study of 'lives in the balance' demonstrates clearly, however, that simple documentation of the facts about drug inject-ing or sexual behaviour is not enough. A true understanding of the lifestyles and the problems of the people concerned is crucial. Their actions and attitudes can be comprehended only in the context of their particular circumstances. This is a vivid and compassionate account of a culture hidden to most people, in which lives are now put at risk of HIV infection. Insights such as this are essential for the provision of effective intervention and help.

Mildred Blaxter
Coordinator, ESRC Programme
of Research on Behavioural
Aspects of HIV/AIDS

Preface

Few diseases have highlighted the interaction between human behaviour, health and disease as AIDS has done. Today, ten years after the first cases of AIDS were reported, the need to characterize the complex interaction of psychosocial and cultural factors that place individuals, families and communities at risk of HIV and AIDS has become imperative. In the absence of more precise information, it will continue to be difficult to address the special needs of individuals and communities with respect to prevention, care and treatment.

To date AIDS has primarily affected individuals with specific sexual and drug use behaviour patterns known to facilitate the transmission of HIV. For a variety of reasons, many of these behaviours and practices have traditionally been socially marginalized. In many societies they are punishable by law and, in recent decades, have become increasingly covert. Drug abuse, especially drug injecting behaviour, has been typical of this trend. Partially as a result of its covert nature, but also because of methodological difficulties involved in studying it, little has been traditionally known about illicit drug injecting, the range of practices involved, and the magnitude of the health and social problems associated with them.

Why and under what circumstances individuals inject drugs, why they share needles, syringes and other injecting equipment, and why they do or do not participate in schemes designed to reduce the risks of HIV continue to be critical issues about which more needs to be known. People who inject drugs have also been singled out in many parts of the world as a source of sexual transmission of HIV to their partners, irrespective of whether they too inject drugs, and to their offspring. The need for interventions designed to promote safer sex, including the regular use of

condoms, has become a priority concern within most HIV/AIDS programmes designed for injecting drug users.

Now at the end of the first decade of the AIDS pandemic, it is also
evident that injecting drug users in some parts of the world have already
been infected with HIV. Many have developed AIDS. The implications of
this for health care and social support are diverse and complex. Problems
associated with 'living with HIV and AIDS' are often exacerbated by the
life-styles associated with drug injecting and vice-versa. How these issues
can be satisfactorily dealt with in a way that allows the medical and psychosocial needs of people to be comprehensively met depends upon how much
knowledge can be accrued on the intricacies of the problem in different
social situations.

How social support can be mobilized in order to reduce the health risks
associated with drug injecting and needle and syringe sharing is similarly a
function of how much can be learned about individual and group coping
strategies. Families, friends and others are all, in one way or another,
affected. Their capacity and willingness to respond constructively to the
needs of people infected with HIV is influenced by local attitudes to drug
abuse and the interaction between drug abusers and other people in the
community.

Lives in the Balance goes far in exploring and explaining some of these
dilemmas. In taking an ethnogaphic approach to drug injecting behaviour
the authors have avoided some of the problems all too often confronted in
survey work, namely of missing the 'small group' dynamics that are essential to any comprehensive understanding of the problem. Instead they have
provided a much needed richness of detailed insight which will provide
health staff and public health planners with a sound base for action. Hope-
fully the research model employed here will be borrowed by others and
used to analyse additional aspects of this relatively new health problem that
is threatening developed and developing countries alike.

Manuel Carballo, PhD, MPH, DSP
Chief of Research and Development
Programme on Substance Abuse
World Health Organization

Acknowledgements

Over the three years we have been working on the research described in this book we have incurred many debts. First and foremost, this study would not have been possible without the help of the many people who were the subjects of our research, those who were injecting drugs and those who were not. For reasons of confidentiality we are unable to identify those people by name, but we are, nevertheless, grateful for the access they allowed us to their lives. Thanks are also due to the many people who helped this research by allowing us access to the various treatment and community settings where young people could be contacted. We would also like to record our thanks to Andrew Boddy, director of the Public Health Research Unit, Sally Macintyre, director of the MRC Medical Sociology Unit and Michael Bloor who were co-grantholders on the project with Neil McKeganey. We owe a special debt to Michael Bloor who helped us in many ways, not least in sharing the many late nights of fieldwork during the prostitute phase of our work. He also nudged us into looking at the work of Alfred Schutz which proved invaluable in understanding needle and syringe sharing. Other colleagues have also helped us at various stages of our work. In particular we would like to thank: Sarah Cunningham-Burley, Professor Raymond Illsley, David Goldberg and Harry Watson; Dr Elizabeth Wilson of the Glasgow Family Planning Clinic; Dr Laurence Gruer of the Greater Glasgow Health Board; and representatives of Strathclyde Regional Police who also helped us in this research. This study was funded by the Economic and Social Research Council as part of their AIDS iniative. We would particularly like to acknowledge the work of Mildred Blaxter in co-ordinating that initiative. Finally, Margaret Seaforth, Rita Dobbs and Karen Hegyi provided secretarial support to our project.

The Public Health Research Unit is funded by the Chief Scientist Office of the Scottish Home and Health Department and the Greater Glasgow Health Board. The opinions expressed in this book are not necessarily those of the Scottish Home and Health Department.

Introduction

Injecting drug abusers have the lowest status of any of those deemed to be at risk of HIV infection. They are the least powerful, least articulate and probably most easily manipulated of all the groups exposed to HIV infection. They are also the group many people fear the most. Illicit drug injectors, it is widely thought, are the ones most likely to generate the further spread of the virus to the wider, non-drug injecting population through sexual intercourse. Such a fear is rooted in a profound ignorance of drug injectors. There is also a perception that drug injectors are all alike; however, the denial that individual drug injectors may differ by more than they have in common amounts to a form of cultural stereotyping.

In this book we have tried to avoid such stereotyping by looking in detail at those aspects of illicit drug injectors' behaviour known to be associated with the spread of HIV infection. Our intention has been to study drug injectors in much the same way that an ethnographer would study a foreign culture. We have sought to try and understand the culture that drug injectors share and to place their behaviour in relation to HIV within that culture. It has been our belief throughout the research on which this book is based that efforts aimed at reducing drug injectors' risks of becoming infected with HIV are likely to be more successful where they are based on a fuller understanding of drug injectors' behaviour. Ours then is an ethnography of drug injectors' risk behaviour, but with the specific intention of identifying information that will be relevant to designing services and other interventions that might reduce the spread of HIV infection between drug injectors. At the end of each of the main chapters in this book we highlight the policy and service implications of our work.

In Chapter 1 we look at the existing literature on the worldwide spread of AIDS and HIV, and the particular role drug injectors have played in that spread. We look at the very different patterns of HIV spread in different cities and countries, and consider some of the explanations offered for those differences. We also look at the situation for women and the increasing importance of paediatric HIV. The three broad areas of HIV risk behaviour on which we concentrate are the sharing of used needles and syringes, sexual contact and prostitution. We also look at the overlap between each of these areas.

In Chapter 2 our focus shifts from a concern with the worldwide spread of HIV amongst drug injectors to look at the particular area of Glasgow where many of our contacts with drug injectors were established. Our intention in this chapter is to try to convey something of what life is like more generally in an area where drug injecting has become commonplace in the last decade. This description sets the scene for much of what we go on to say about drug injectors' lifestyles and HIV-related risk behaviour.

In Chapter 3 we look at what is probably the single most important factor in the spread of HIV infection amongst drug injectors, namely, the sharing of used needles and syringes. We show how such sharing may be influenced by aspects of the wider culture, as well as by aspects of the drug injector's own shared culture. We draw upon the work of Alfred Schutz to show how sharing arises out of the everyday situations in which drugs are being injected.

In Chapter 4 our attention shifts from needle and syringe sharing to the question of heterosexual transmission of HIV infection. In their attitudes towards sex and condom use drug injectors are not greatly different from the majority of others and so this chapter has a rather broader focus than a concern with drug injectors alone.

In Chapter 5 we concentrate specifically upon male and female prostitution. From studies throughout Europe and North America it has been shown that at least some individuals use prostitution as a way of financing their drug injecting; whether such prostitution will represent an important pathway for the spread of HIV infection is looked at in this chapter.

In Chapter 6 we focus on the experiences of those drug injectors who are already living with the diagnosis of being HIV positive. We look at the situations in which they found out that they were HIV positive and their reactions to the diagnosis. We also look at the way in which being positive has influenced virtually every facet of their lives, from their relationships with others, to starting a family, to sex and to their hopes for their future.

Finally, in Chapter 7 we try and draw the various strands of our work together and make some assessment as to what the future might hold for many of the people whose lives we have portrayed in this book.

Chapter 1

Drug injectors and the worldwide epidemic of HIV infection

It is a measure of the seriousness of the HIV/AIDS epidemic that, even in the short space of time since the virus was discovered, a vast and burgeoning body of literature on the subject has emerged. In this chapter we will review a portion of that literature.

We look first at the global impact of HIV and AIDS especially within those countries which have a high prevalence of HIV infection. Since drug injectors form the focus of this book we look specifically at the existing literature in relation to the three broad areas of risk behaviours associated with drug injectors: needle and syringe sharing; the practice of unprotected sex; and the use of prostitution as a means of financially supporting a drug habit.

The global impact of HIV and AIDS

Cases of HIV infection and AIDS have now been reported the world over. Reports from the World Health Organization (WHO) clearly show that HIV infection has continued to spread rapidly during the last decade. The WHO now estimate that by the year 2000, 25–30 million men, women and children will be infected with HIV. Cumulative totals of AIDS cases reported to the WHO as of 1 September 1990 were 283,010 from 157 countries. However, this figure is acknowledged to under-represent the actual number of AIDS cases. It has been estimated that there may be as many as 1.2 million men, women and children in the world with AIDS (*Answer* 1990a).

Even though HIV and AIDS are now prevalent worldwide, the pattern of spread remains highly variable both within and between populations. Three broad factors are thought to account for the variability. First, the year in which the virus was introduced into an area clearly has an important bearing on the degree to which HIV infection is spread within a population. Differences in cumulative AIDS case rates are, at least in part, thought to be attributable to differences in the time when epidemic spread of the virus began (Sato *et al.* 1989). It is generally accepted, for example, that the HIV epidemic began in Europe approximately two years later than it did in the United States and that this is reflected in differences in the number of AIDS cases between the two areas.

Second, an accurate assessment of the spread of HIV and AIDS over time depends on the availability of complete and accurate global AIDS statistics. AIDS case detection and reporting are not, however, consistent across all countries and continents. In some industrialized countries it is estimated that approximately 80 per cent of cases are detected and reported, whilst for some African nations this figure drops to about 10 per cent (Chin and Mann 1988).

The third and most important factor used to explain the uneven distribution of HIV infection across different populations is that those behaviour patterns which have resulted in the majority of HIV infections, principally sexual intercourse and injecting drug use, themselves vary within and across populations.

As a result of the different patterns of spread of HIV infection within different countries, the World Health Organization has created a classificatory schema for categorizing different countries and different geographical regions. Pattern I type areas are primarily western industrialized nations where HIV is predominantly found amongst homosexual/bisexual men and injecting drug users. The numbers of people infected through heterosexual sex alone are still low. As men form the majority of those infected there are relatively small numbers of children with paediatric AIDS.

Pattern II type areas have a quite different epidemiology. These countries are primarily in sub-Saharan Africa and some parts of the Caribbean. HIV is widespread throughout these areas and can exceed 25 per cent in some urban areas (Sato *et al.* 1989). Transmission of HIV mostly occurs through unprotected heterosexual sex, although a significant number of people in pattern II areas are still becoming infected through contaminated blood or blood products. Since there are approximately as many women as men who are HIV infected, there is high prevalence of paediatric AIDS.

Pattern III areas have few cases of HIV/AIDS to date which may be a reflection of the comparatively late introduction of HIV infection into these areas. However, low levels of HIV infection can change dramatically over a very short time, particularly if recent sharp increases in the numbers becoming HIV infected in Bangkok and northern India are anything to go by (Sato *et al.* 1989). The WHO schema, however, is not fixed and it is certain that countries as well as whole areas are likely to move between patterns as their epidemic of HIV unfolds. In Latin America, for example,

the virus was initially found in urban homosexual/bisexual men and injecting drug users. In the last half of the 1980s, however, an increasing number
of infections have been heterosexually transmitted. Similarly, as more
women have become infected so there has also been an increase in cases
of paediatric AIDS. Thus, Latin America is defined as being in transition
from pattern I to pattern II and is now classified as having a separate
epidemiologic pattern (pattern I/II).

Injecting drug use and HIV infection

In many of the developed countries the early 1980s saw an explosion in
numbers of young people illicitly using injectable drugs (Stimson 1987).
Within Britain and elsewhere the new drug users of the 1980s were largely
to be found in inner city areas characterized by widespread socio-economic
deprivation (Parker et al. 1988; Stoneburner et al. 1990), typically they were
young and male, and heroin was their first choice of drug. At the same time
as injecting became an increasingly popular means of administering drugs,
so too HIV infection was silently spreading within drug injecting populations. Data from various cities in North America and Europe indicate that
HIV has been present in populations of drug injectors since 1977 in New
York (Thomas et al. 1988), 1979 in Northern Italy (Tempesta and di
Giannantonio 1988) and 1983 in Edinburgh (Robertson et al. 1986).

The rapidity with which HIV can spread once established within populations of drug injectors is well illustrated by the situation in New York
City, Edinburgh and Milan. These cities have all experienced epidemic
spread of the virus resulting in known seroprevalence rates of over 50 per
cent in injecting drug users (Des Jarlais et al. 1987). In Bangkok, Thailand,
HIV seroprevalence rates shot from approximately 15.6 per cent in 1988 to
42.7 per cent in 1989 (Vanichseni et al. 1990). The same startling increases
have been recently reported in Manipur, North India, an area bordering
the Golden Triangle (Burma, Laos and Thailand) where large quantities of
heroin are produced. Routine testing of injecting drug users through 1989
to 1990 in Manipur showed that where there was no known HIV infection
in 1989, by June 1990 the HIV seroprevalence rate was 54 per cent (Naik et
al. 1991).

Even though HIV infection has the potential to spread rapidly within
drug injecting populations its spread has not been geographically uniform.
Britain is a case in point. Despite a large overall population of drug
injectors, HIV seroprevalence is thought to be low in all British cities
with the exception of Edinburgh and more recently, London. In Edinburgh, approximately 51 per cent of known injectors are thought to be
HIV positive. It is important to stress, however, that the figure of 51 per
cent is based upon samples of injectors recruited at treatment sites who

may not be representative of drug injectors as a whole in that city. The situation in Edinburgh is similar only to New York City (Des Jarlais and Friedman 1990), Barcelona (Muga et al. 1990) and Milan in Northern Italy (Tempesta and Di Giannantonio 1990).

The uneven distribution of HIV infection among drug injectors can be highlighted by the contrasting fortunes of Edinburgh and Glasgow. Despite being approximately 50 miles apart these two cities have very marked differences in the prevalence of HIV infection. Whilst over half of known Edinburgh injectors are HIV seropositive, only 1.4 per cent of Glasgow resident drug injectors in a recent study were found to have antibodies for HIV (Haw et al. 1991). A number of possible explanations have been put forward to explain the differences in seroprevalence rates.

The date of introduction of HIV infection into local populations of drug injectors might go some way towards explaining differences in the numbers of people who are HIV infected. Whereas HIV infection was detected in 1983 in Edinburgh, in Glasgow its earliest appearance is reportedly 1985 (Follett et al. 1986).

Another factor influencing differences in HIV rates relates to the frequency with which unsterile injecting equipment is used and the numbers of people involved. Findings from a number of studies indicate a strong association between the frequency of needle and syringe sharing, and HIV seropositivity (Des Jarlais et al. 1986; Marmor et al. 1987). Robertson and his colleagues showed that in Edinburgh larger numbers of injectors were often present when needles and syringes were shared than was the case in Glasgow. Gatherings of between 10 and 20 injectors were apparently not uncommon in 1983 (Robertson et al. 1986).

This pattern of behaviour was not reported to occur among Glasgow injectors (Follett et al. 1986), perhaps in part because the Glasgow injectors did not experience the same difficulties in obtaining sterile injecting equipment as was reportedly the case in Edinburgh (Robertson 1990). This continues to be the case in New York City and New Jersey as a whole, where possession of injecting equipment is an arrestable offence (Friedman et al. 1990a).

It should be noted, however, that the above explanations as to why one city has high levels of HIV infection among drug injectors whilst another has not, are not wholly adequate. If it were solely a matter of availability of sterile needles and syringes, for example, there would be little HIV infection among drug injectors in Italy where injecting equipment has been widely available for many years (Tempesta and Di Giannantonio 1990). Furthermore, in Glasgow, although needles and syringes can be obtained from selected pharmacies or from needle exchanges located in areas where large numbers of drug injectors are known to live, our own study found a good deal of needle sharing still occurring even within those areas (McKeganey et al. 1989).

Needle sharing

Since it first became apparent that HIV was present in populations of drug injectors, numerous studies have demonstrated a strong link between the shared use of unsterile injecting equipment and HIV infection. These studies are geographically widespread and include the United States (Chaisson *et al.* 1987; Des Jarlais and Friedman 1987; Battjes *et al.* 1989), Italy (Rezza *et al.* 1989) and Scotland (Robertson *et al.* 1986). More recently, studies in Thailand (Vanichseni *et al.* 1990) and North India (Naik *et al.* 1991) have again demonstrated the strong association between shared use of unsterile needles and HIV infection.

In looking at the relationship between needle sharing and HIV infection the social dimensions of drug injectors' behaviour needs to be taken into adequate account. Only a handful of studies have systematically turned their attention to needle sharing as a social behaviour having social meaning for those concerned. This includes a San Francisco based study conducted long before HIV and AIDS was known about (Howard and Borges 1970). This work very clearly showed that needle sharing was a socially situated response to local circumstances and social ties between injectors.

Howard and Borges found that a large number of the injectors they interviewed were sharing injecting equipment. This was in spite of a high level of awareness of the risks of contracting blood borne infections such as hepatitis B. The reasons given for sharing related not only to lack of availability of clean equipment, but more broadly to the social context of a drug injecting lifestyle. They found that sharing needles and syringes was culturally expected among injectors, and on a personal level was an expression of close relationships or friendships. They also found that large numbers of injectors were using drugs in the company of others, both because drug use was viewed as a social event and because the presence of others conferred a sense of protection in the event of such occurrences as drug overdose. Women were much more likely to inject in the company of others; the majority of them did not, in fact, inject themselves, but were injected by men.

More recently, researchers in the United States (Des Jarlais *et al.* 1986; Friedman *et al.* 1990a) and in Amsterdam (Grund *et al.* 1991) have demonstrated that needle and syringe sharing has a continuing importance amongst drug injectors even if it occurs less frequently today than in the past.

Other work also points to the value of looking at patterns of interaction rather than individual risk behaviour patterns. Friedman and his colleagues (1989), for example, have found differences in the behaviour of new injectors compared to that of older more experienced injectors. They found that the younger, relatively inexperienced injectors were engaging in higher levels of risk behaviour between themselves than was the case amongst the more experienced injectors (Grund and his associates similarly report this in a study of injecting drug users in Holland, 1991). Despite this, however, few of the recent initiates into injecting drug use were HIV positive. Friedman and his colleagues suggest that the explanation for this may lie in the social relationships between injectors. They found that those individuals who have only recently begun injecting tend, at first, to inject (and share needles and syringes) with other initiates whose exposure to HIV at this time would be limited. However, as these injectors become more experienced so they come into greater contact with a wider spectrum of injectors. As HIV is prevalent among the more experienced injectors, the likelihood of coming into contact with HIV infection increases as they become more immersed in the drug using culture and extend their contacts with its members.

Where needle sharing has been examined in some detail it is clear that it is very much a social behaviour with such factors as *who* shares, with *whom* and how *frequently* being social processes that are as likely to influence the direction of HIV spread as are issues such as the availability of injecting equipment. In Chapter 3 we look at the social processes of needle and syringe sharing in greater detail.

Drug injectors and the heterosexual spread of HIV infection

Drug injectors are thought to face their greatest risk of becoming HIV infected through the use of unsterile needles and syringes. To a degree, however, this is likely to be an artefact of the current practice of the American Centers for Disease Control and the British Public Health Laboratory Service to classify individuals under a single risk category even though multiple risk practices might be involved. Decisions on the classification of cases where more than one risk factor is present are made on the basis of which factor was thought most likely to have resulted in infection (Bloor *et al.* 1991a). Increasingly, however, it is recognized that the risk of heterosexually transmitted HIV is by no means negligible and should be taken seriously (Cowan *et al.* 1989; Robertson and Skidmore 1989).

The potential for heterosexual transmission of the virus is evident in a population which is predominantly heterosexually active and where raised levels of HIV have been identified (Des Jarlais *et al.* 1988). Perhaps the best evidence for this potential lies in the spread of HIV to heterosexuals with no known risk factor beyond sexual contact with someone whose behaviour is a high risk for HIV infection (Public Health Laboratory Service (PHLS) Collaborative Study Group 1989; Stoneburner *et al.* 1990).

It has been suggested that differences in the likelihood of an individual becoming HIV positive as a result of coming into contact with the virus may be related to the presence of co-factors such as sexually transmitted diseases (Brunet *et al.* 1987). The degree to which co-factors are influencing the transmission of HIV may go some considerable way towards explaining global variations in HIV spread.

Heterosexual spread of HIV infection in North America and Europe appears to have a relatively distinctive pattern. First, the overwhelming majority of cases of heterosexually acquired HIV appear to have arisen as a result of sexual contact with an individual at risk of HIV, usually through injecting drug use, (Shapiro *et al.* 1989; Norman *et al.* 1990). There is, as yet, little evidence to suggest the wider spread of infection (Chaisson *et al.* 1990). Second, the available data on heterosexual transmission indicate that, proportionately, women may be at greater risk of acquiring the virus than men (Cohen *et al.* 1989).

Recent reports from the Communicable Diseases (Scotland) Unit would seem to be a case in point. Although there are cases of men acquiring the virus heterosexually in Scotland, their numbers remain small (58 out of the total 1242 HIV positive men, 4.6 per cent). Amongst HIV positive women however the situation is different, 96 out of 501 (19.2 per cent) having been infected heterosexually. The main transmission route is believed to be sexual contact with a male partner whose behaviour carries a risk of HIV transmission (*Answer* 1990b). Most often, the partner of the infected person has been an injecting drug user. This situation is also true for Europe and North America (Brunet *et al.* 1987; Chaisson *et al.* 1990).

There are two possible explanations for this trend. The first is related to gender differences in the social structure of injecting drug use and the second appears to concern sex-related differences in physiological suscep-tibility to the virus. It is now widely accepted that the absolute majority of injectors are male (McKeganey *et al.* 1989; Frischer 1991). Furthermore the majority of these men have non-drug injecting girlfriends with whom they are sexually active (Donoghoe *et al.* 1989; Robertson and Skidmore 1989). The tendency for male drug injectors to have female partners who do not inject drugs may play a significant part in predicting the likely direction of HIV spread from drug injectors to the general non-drug injecting hetero-sexual population. Additionally, since HIV seroprevalence is greater in men, a woman is more likely than a man to have an infected heterosexual partner (*MMWR* 1989). However, it would appear that there are other factors influencing women's increased susceptibility to the virus. There is evidence from a number of studies (Nicolosi 1990; Stoneburner *et al.* 1990) that sexual transmission is more likely to occur from male to female than female to male. Women are not only more likely to be exposed to the virus, but that exposure is also more likely to result in infection.

Women using drugs may be considered as doubly at risk of HIV through their drug use and through their sexual contacts, which are predominantly with men also injecting drugs. This may be illustrated by reference to the situation in Glasgow where 54 per cent of drug injectors identified as

HIV antibody positive are women. Despite the fact that many more men than women are drug injectors, it is predominantly drug injecting women who are HIV infected (*Answer* 1990b).

Whilst attention has been drawn to the probable differences between women and men's experiences of HIV (Coxon and Carballo 1989; Sato *et al.* 1989), few studies have systematically explored these differences. Relatively little is known, for example, about the natural history of HIV infection in women (Chin 1990) or, indeed, the special needs of women, particularly where childbirth is concerned (Selwyn *et al.* 1990). Since the numbers of women with HIV infection are slowly but surely increasing, attention has begun to focus more specifically on HIV positive women (Norman *et al.* 1990). This shift in attention away from an almost exclusive concern with men may, in fact, reflect the changes in the course of the HIV epidemic. The incidence of HIV amongst men began to level off in the mid-1980s whilst the incidence of HIV amongst women began to increase at about this time (Chin 1990).

In some areas where the prevalence of HIV amongst drug injectors is high, for instance New York City and Connecticut, HIV seroprevalence rates in men and women are similar, although more men than women are infected because there are higher absolute numbers of men injectors than women (Shapiro *et al.* 1989). In the United Kingdom, women of all risk categories currently account for about one-third of new cases in Scotland and one sixth of new cases in England, Wales and Northern Ireland (Norman *et al.* 1990). Importantly, four-fifths of British HIV positive women are of reproductive age, which is similar to the situation in the United States where 85 per cent of HIV positive women are of an age where reproduction is possible (Shapiro *et al.* 1989). This, in itself, raises a whole series of medical, social, moral and ethical issues which need to be addressed.

The majority of HIV positive women in Europe and North America are either themselves injecting drug users or have partners with a history of injecting drug use (Peckham and Newell 1990). Female injectors are known to have a high rate of pregnancies, many of which are unplanned as a result of irregular contraceptive use (Cohen *et al.* 1989; Selwyn *et al.* 1990). As the incidence of HIV infection among women increases so, too, we may expect an increase in the numbers of HIV infected babies being born to these women. This is already happening in areas of high HIV seroprevalence; for example, in the Bronx, New York City, the HIV prevalence in women giving birth is 1 in 43 (Novick *et al.* 1989).

At an earlier stage in the epidemic it was estimated that the risk of an HIV infected mother giving birth to an HIV positive child was approximately 50 per cent. On the basis of information from more recent studies these estimates have now been downwardly revised (Pizzo 1989, Andiman *et al.* 1990). In France, for example, a prospective study of 117 infants showed only one-third of infants as likely to show evidence of HIV/AIDS by 18 months (Blanche *et al.* 1989). In New York City the current rate of perinatal transmission is 29 per cent once the maternal antibodies have been replaced by the baby's own antibodies (Joseph 1989). However, the most recently published findings from ten European centres, based on 600 children born to HIV infected mothers and followed up until at least 18 months after birth is a transmission rate of just 13 per cent (European Collaborative Study 1991).

Even this comparatively low risk of passing on HIV infection to an unborn child may, however, be regarded as unacceptably high in some circles. It should be borne in mind that the issue of childbirth is a highly sensitive one and tightly bound with personal values, prevailing cultural expectations and social circumstances (Arras 1990; Levine and Dubler 1990). It cannot be expected that an HIV diagnosis will necessarily result in a woman terminating her pregnancy. This was demonstrated in a recent study which found that knowledge of the HIV state did not determine whether the woman terminated the pregnancy or continued it to full term. Personal and/or social factors were also significant in determining the outcome (Selwyn *et al.* 1990). The whole issue of women transmitting HIV infection to their unborn children is both powerfully emotive and inevitably controversial. HIV positive women face difficult personal and moral dilemmas in making decisions about reproduction. Expected increases in the number of HIV infected women further underlines the importance of addressing these issues as well as providing for the particular constellation of needs which these women and their children are likely to have. We look at the issue of heterosexual transmission of HIV in greater detail in Chapter 4 and in Chapter 5 we look at some of the ways in which a diagnosis of being HIV positive can influence the decision to start a family.

The association between HIV infection, prostitution and drug injecting

Perhaps the first point to make here is that there is no consistent global pattern in the association between prostitution and AIDS (Padian 1988). In sub-Saharan Africa prostitution appears to have played a significant part in the spread of HIV infection (D'Costa *et al.* 1985; Piot *et al.* 1987). However, within Europe and North America a very different picture seems to have emerged as prostitution does *not* appear to be playing a significant role in the transmission of HIV (Cohen *et al.* 1989; Chaisson *et al.* 1990). In fact, early reports from the United States showed similar rates of HIV infection among prostitutes as for the total population in each area (*MMWR* 1987). That prostitution in these areas does not appear to have played such a significant role in HIV transmission to date does not, of course, mean that this will always be the case. Recent reports from some North American cities showing an association between the use of crack cocaine and high risk sexual behaviour clearly give considerable cause for concern (Golden *et al*. 1990; Weissman *et al*. 1990). Similarly, particular concern has also been expressed with respect to women who are prostituting in order to finance injecting drug use. Information on the heterosexual spread of HIV infection suggests that unprotected sexual contact with individuals engaging in high risk activities (primarily injecting drug use and unprotected male homosexual intercourse) is a significant risk factor in HIV transmission (Des Jarlais *et al*. 1987; Stoneburner *et al*. 1990). The use of prostitution to finance a drug habit gives rise to concern since raised levels of HIV infection have been identified amongst female drug injecting prostitutes compared to non-drug injecting prostitute women (Tirelli *et al*. 1989; Doerr *et al*. 1990).

Recent research carried out in a number of cities in the United Kingdom and elsewhere suggests that there is considerable overlap between female prostitution and injecting drug use. In London, Day and her colleagues (1988) found that 14 per cent of their sample of female prostitutes were injecting drug users, while in Birmingham, Kinnell (1989) found that 15 per cent of the female prostitutes she contacted were injecting drug users, and Morgan Thomas and her colleagues in Edinburgh found that 28 per cent of the female prostitutes they contacted were injecting drug users (Morgan-Thomas *et al*. 1989).

The significance of the overlap between drug injecting and prostitution can only be assessed in terms of detailed information on such topics as the extent of HIV infection among prostitutes, the extent of needle and syringe sharing between prostitutes, and the frequency of condom use between prostitutes, their clients and their non-paying partners. However, data on these areas are only just beginning to become available. There is a good deal of evidence from North America and Europe showing that prostitute women are using condoms with clients either all or most of the time (McKeganey *et al*. 1990a; van den Hoek *et al*. 1990). It is also apparent, however, that many prostitute women do not use condoms with private, non-paying partners. It may be that many prostitutes are at greater risk of HIV infection from their private partners. These issues are looked at in greater detail in Chapter 6 where we concentrate specifically on the link between prostitution and HIV infection; we also examine the relationships prostitutes establish with clients and examine some of the ways in which these relationships may hinder or facilitate HIV risk reduction.

In this chapter we have outlined current thinking among researchers on issues relating to drug injectors' risks of HIV infection. In the following chapters we look at our own work on drug injectors' risk behaviour. To set the scene for our description of drug injectors' risk behaviour it is worth describing in some detail the local area where many of our contacts with drug injectors were established. As we will show in the chapter on needle sharing, much of the risk behaviour we identified could be explained in terms of the broader culture in the local area.

Chapter 2

The social context: Glasgow

Introduction

Many AIDS-related studies have shown a tendency to focus upon behaviours known to transmit HIV infection in isolation from their social context. Although understandable, there is some danger in this since HIV risk behaviour patterns, such as needle and syringe sharing or unprotected sexual contact, do not occur within a vacuum, but as part of a much wider context of human relationships. To understand why individuals share injecting equipment, for example, it is necessary to understand something about the meaning of social obligations and social ties between people within an area.

A second, related tendency in behavioural studies of HIV infection is to focus attention only on those individuals with certain risk behaviour patterns, for example drug injectors or male homosexuals. This gives the impression that these individuals are somehow entirely separate from other people, and subject to quite unique pressures, norms and beliefs. Although much of what we say in subsequent chapters is specific to drug injectors' HIV-related risk behaviour, in this chapter we will take a rather broader approach and try and convey something of what life is like more generally in the area where many of our contacts were established.

Any description of an area or its people, however, can offer only a partial view; our own description, no less than that of others, is influenced by our particular standpoint as researchers carrying out a study of drug injectors' risk behaviour. For this reason we have chosen to interweave our description of the local area with a description of our own work as researchers and participant observers.

Identifying an area and initial impressions

In the early 1980s Glasgow, along with many other British cities, seems to have undergone a local epidemic of heroin use. In 1985 there were an estimated 5000 injectors in the city (Haw 1985). That figure is now believed to have increased to an estimated 9500 injectors out of a total population of approximately 1.2 million (Frischer *et al.* 1991).

The area we chose to concentrate upon was typical of many parts of the city where there are large numbers of drug injectors. It is an area characterized by severe physical and social deprivation. Visually, it is a depressing area, many of the tenement blocks stand empty and boarded up, there are few trees and few amenities which have not been vandalized. Despite recent efforts to halt the physical deterioration of the area by renovating houses and improving the general outlook, marked social deprivation produced by low incomes and high unemployment remains untackled, and indeed has deepened in consequence of government cuts in social support throughout the 1980s.

At the time of the 1981 census over 50 per cent of people aged between 16 and 24 were unemployed, this percentage being only marginally lower for people aged between 25 and 49. There were large numbers of single parents and large families in the area, and overcrowding was a common feature of many households. It is a further indication of the poor socio-economic fabric of the area that 93 per cent of households did not have ownership of a car.

With the advent of widespread drug use throughout the 1980s the situation has, if anything, deteriorated further. The evidence of injecting drug use lies everywhere, many of the stairwells of derelict tenements are used for the purpose of injecting drugs, and are littered with the associated paraphernalia of syringes, drug capsules and water bottles.

To broaden our contacts beyond drug injectors we spent many evenings during our year of fieldwork in the area attending the local community centre. In addition, one of us was attached to a local Intermediate Treatment group (IT) run by the social work department for young people with difficulties either at school or at home. We also ran a series of discussion groups with pupils aged between 14 and 16 attending the two local schools, and spent an extended period of time literally on the streets talking to local people.

To contact drug injectors we carried out semi-structured interviews within a local retail pharmacy which sold injecting equipment, within the nearby needle exchange and within an out-patient clinic of Glasgow's infectious diseases hospital. In this last setting we were able to interview 26 drug injectors who had already been diagnosed as HIV positive. Additionally, we carried out interviews with over 40 injecting drug users who were temporarily resident in a variety of drug detoxification centres within the city. To look at the overlap between prostitution, injecting drug use and HIV-related risk behaviour we carried out street interviews with 208 female prostitutes and 32 male prostitutes who worked the city's 'red light' areas. This aspect of our work is described in greater detail in Chapter 6.

The area we chose to focus upon and where most of our contacts with drug injectors and others not injecting drugs lived, was characterized by many harsh contrasts. The physical desolation and dilapidation of many of the buildings was often reflected in people's own descriptions of their surroundings. In the field-note below, and in all subsequent field-notes, we have altered individuals' names and certain biographical features to maintain the anonymity of our research contacts.

We were standing with Steven when he commented 'There's a bad feel to this place, a really bad feel.' I asked if he meant the street we were standing in. 'No no the whole area, there's a fuckin' great black cloud hangin' over this place, I hate it. I hate this place but I could never leave it, the most I've ever left it for was 6 months when I was in the army.'

(Streetwork field-note)

We passed a group of teenage boys, one of whom looked over at us and shouted 'you writing a book about this place?' Neil said we were. They asked what it was about. Neil replied, 'Life round here, what it's like to grow up here.' One said, 'what like, about the vandalism?' One of the boys who was walking ahead turned round and commented 'It's a dump, put that in your book, full of junkies.'

(Streetwork field-note)

At the same time, however, people were often fiercely loyal to their area, defending it verbally and often physically from the merest hint of criticism from outsiders. The existence of strong local loyalties and rivalries between localities appears to have a long history in Glasgow (Patrick 1973). Many people stated that although they were safe in their area, this safety could not be guaranteed in other areas where they were not known.

It was an area where the social obligations of friendship seemed to exist as a kind of supra-ordinate moral code; to defend one's own was what mattered.

Jerry arrived at the Community Centre in the middle of the evening and wandered over to our group. This led to a long discussion orchestrated by Mickey as to whether he (Jerry) would have let the guys into the Centre if the community worker had said they weren't allowed in. 'Would you have opened the doors if she had said no?' 'But she didn't' Jerry answered defensively 'She wasn't saying that.' Mickey persisted, 'No but would you if she had? If you wouldn't have done you're not one of us.' It was interesting listening to this because even though the situation was entirely hypothetical the issue of Jerry's allegiance to the group was very real. I was reminded in this of the way in which none of them will ever purchase a cup of tea without asking all of the others if they also want a cup. On one occasion I was pulled up for not having supplied chocolate biscuits when I bought the tea. The sense of group solidarity is seen as uppermost even in things as mundane as this.

(Community centre)

Despite such an emphasis on group solidarity there were very few overt displays of tenderness or affection between local people. On the contrary, relationships between local people often had what seemed to us to be a hard, antagonistic edge to them.

Nicky (non-injector) asked me if I wanted to go back to his Dad's house where we could look for the address of one of the lads that had moved temporarily to London. We left the Centre, crossed the street and entered what I first took to be a derelict block. Nicky strode down the dark corridor and I tried to keep up with him whilst wary of stumbling over any objects in the dark. Nicky unlocked the front door to one of the flats and we entered. The place was incredibly small and stuffed full of furniture such that one could hardly move. Nicky began an immediate and seemingly frantic search through drawers and old boxes in what I guessed would be a fruitless search. At this point I heard someone else entering the block. Nicky, perhaps sensing my unease, said 'och, it's a crazy junkie. If he comes in here he'll hit you and you'll get AIDS.' He laughed gleefully and returned to his search. There was a knock at the door, Nicky called out, 'Who's that?' 'It's your mother' the person on the other side of the door answered. Nicky turned to me 'Whit the fuck does she want?' His mother entered the flat. She was small, frail and rather tired looking. The two immediately began arguing. Nicky offered her £5 in what I took to be repayment of a debt but when his mother asked him where his father was he snapped back 'what d'ye want to know for, gonnae tap him for money as well?' Later, when Nicky's father arrived, the mother asked if he would go and get her some cans of beer. She later turned to Nicky and me, flipped open her purse (full of money) and said 'I've nae need to tap him for money,' even though she had just done so. The family dynamics in the flat seemed entirely strange to me, with everyone throwing insults at each other.

(Streetwork field-note)

A group of five drug injectors were joined by another guy and soon after an argument began. It appeared to be about a young lad who'd been ripped off by one of them. The argument continued until a glass bottle was forcefully thrown at the offending party's head as he walked away. He moved just out of the way as it smashed heavily into the road and splintered everywhere. He then came back to the guy who'd thrown it and continued to argue but somehow after that it'd lost its violent edge and the subject was dropped.

(Streetwork field-note)

Although many local relationships had this hard edge, it frequently seemed as if this was more a matter of their surface appearance rather than their deeper nature. Antagonistic sniping seemed to have become an accepted way of relating to others. This is not to suggest that there were no occasions when such aggressiveness did not signal more deep-seated feelings:

We were sitting on the tenement steps talking to four people when the sister of one of the guys we were with (Malcolm) opened one of the upstairs windows and shouted out that she didn't want housebreakers on her step. There was a lot of shouted insults and accusations flying thick and fast. Fitzy shouted back 'who the fuck you calling a housebreaker you midden? I don't need to do that, I do the creep'. I asked what the creep was and Malcolm said it was stealing out of hotel rooms. 'I can earn three ton doin' that, I'm no a housebreaker.' Malcolm's sister continued 'I bet youse the one that steals weans toys an' all, and it's probably youse that's been stealin' clothes off washin' lines.' Malcolm interjected, 'no, that's John.' She turned on him saying 'And I suppose he's the only one doin' it is he?' While the two of them were arguing everyone else stood apart from them and carried on as normal, although we were all listening. Now and again Malcolm would comment to us that she really could exercise her lungs but nobody participated or even seemed particularly perturbed by it. Fitzy commented to Malcolm 'if she doesn't shut up soon I'm goin' tae slap her face and I don't care what you say.' As he turned to leave he said 'It's a shame I cannae get ma sister up from the Cross, she'd gie you a doin'. When he returned he showed us an axe head tucked in his trousers, 'that's for her, if she gets cheeky again.'

(Streetwork field-note)

In contrast to many of the other rows and antagonisms between local people this incident seemed potentially more dangerous. It is interesting to note that none of the assembled group felt the need to intervene. However, when Malcolm was later asked about the argument he had clearly assessed the situation and what action he was prepared to take:

Neil asked what would Malcolm have done if Fitzy had slapped his sister, Malcolm dismissed the probability 'would he fuck, I'd have battered him before he'd done that . . . see when he brought that axe back, that was just show, he wouldnae have done anything.'

(Streetwork field-note)

This incident is also illustrative of other features of the local area. Even though Fitzy and the other members of our group were drug injectors it was not this that drew the woman's wrath, but the possibility that one of them had been breaking into local people's flats; it was this latter, not the drug use that was regarded as socially unacceptable. In Fitzy's defence he asserts that everybody knows that he is not a housebreaker, but someone who does 'the creep'. Stealing from anonymous others in hotels was deemed socially acceptable in a way in which stealing from one's own people was not. One can see here the importance attached to local ties between people.

The distinction between legitimate and illegitimate wrongdoing was also characteristic of the area and was evident, for example, in the widespread buying and selling of stolen goods. Food, and clothing as well as expensive electrical items were all being bought and sold on the informal market on a daily basis. Shoplifting was not a marginal activity so much as a fully fledged parallel economy, seemingly involving anybody and everybody:

Terry (drug injector) regaled us with a story of a recent shoplifting episode when he and his mates had visited a large store in the city centre and had stolen a number of expensive women's quilted jackets. They had been chased out of the shop by store detectives and he had only managed to get away by jumping on a local bus travelling to this area. An old lady on the bus had offered Terry a couple of large plastic bags in which to conceal the jackets – he in repayment sold the lady one for £15.

(Streetwork field-note)

In the middle of the estate a group of young kids were sitting on the kerbside, one of them called over to me. I couldn't make out what he was saying and two of them ran over – one of them removed a pair of spectacles from his face and offered them to me 'They're Burberry, really expensive' and indeed the Burberry price tag for £90 was still attached. I said I didn't want them, that it was a good price and if I heard of anyone who wanted a pair I would let them know. The kid didn't seem overly interested in this rather pathetic evasion but simply returned the spectacles to his face, and ran off.

(Streetwork field-note)

Amongst many of the local people there was a deep seated distrust of official agencies. For example, people generally only spoke in negative terms about the police:

Marina and I sat on the steps of one of the blocks with William and Garry. As we did so a red Vauxhall car drove by with two males inside. William commented that they were plain clothes drug squad officers 'smell 'em a mile away' he said. This latter was somewhat contradicted by William's earlier comment that if the police wanted you they'd batter your door down before any of the neighbours could let out a warning.

(Streetwork field-note)

Earlier in the evening we had watched as two uniformed police appeared round the corner holding a young lad by the lapels and walking him in the direction of the Police Station. We all watched this in silence until Kevin said 'he should have run off to make the fuckers work for their money', and then, with a kind of professional disdain, added: 'they were no' even holdin' him right.'

(Streetwork field-note)

It was not only the police who were seen in this way, the work of social workers and school teachers was also coolly received, and school itself was seen as having little or no value for the local youngsters:

Roddy was talking about the lack of training in the area, 'see round here, you just run wild, you don't bother with school, naebody does. You don't think about anythin' and then it finishes and you're out, that's just how it is round here.'

(Streetwork field-note)

In disciplining young children the adults in the local area often seemed to be remarkably harsh:

We got to the shop, it had no windows and tight security with a man standing in the middle of the shop watching almost every move made. In front of us there was a woman with a child of about 3 years. I found the woman very difficult to age as her face seemed worn. I doubt she was much beyond 25–30 years. She was clearly irritated by her child 'Shut up youse, youse are batterin' ma nerves, shut the fuck up' and then she hit her quite aggressively on the side of the head with the metal shopping basket. I was astounded by this but no one seemed to pay it any mind. The only response was by a woman in front of her who commented to the shop owner, 'she shouldn't swear like that, I wouldnae.' At this everyone laughed at the deliberate irony.

(Streetwork field-note)

Yet at the same time many adults were very protective towards children, modifying their behaviour and what they talked about when in their company:

Sitting at the table chatting with Marina and Helen when Gary, a non-injector in his early twenties arrives in high spirits. He immediately pulls up the waistband of his trousers, prominently revealing the outline of his genitals. All of this is accompanied by Gary calling out to Marina and Helen 'see all this goin' to waste'. Marina walked away and Helen called out 'you're a dirty cunt so you are.' Gary kept this up, deriving enormous entertainment from what he took to be their shocked response. However he stopped all of this when a young girl walked up to the coffee hatch to buy sweets, saying 'I'd better stop this, there's weans about.'

(Community centre)

Ginger who is himself an injector spoke about seeing a small child coming out of a tenement carrying a used needle and syringe with no cap on the needle. Ginger commented that she must have been aware of what it was though because she was holding it just between her fingers. 'I went up to her and took it off her and told her not to touch any more needles she found, I just put it down the stank. Then I went into the tenement close and it was full of dirty works and temazepam caps all over, so I cleaned it up . . . it's all cleaned up now but I bet that by tomorrow it'll be full of caps and works again.'

(Streetwork field-note)

Relationships between local people were most often divided by gender. Within the community centre, for example, the males played pool, chatted, drank coffee and the women chatted amongst themselves. Contact between the two groups seemed pretty minimal, although there was a good deal of taunting:

Marina sat with the women in the coffee area while I hung around with the guys by the pool table. 'I'm bored, I want a new minge.' Nicky announced, 'Know what a minge is Neil, it's Glasgow for fanny.' At this point one of the women walked by to an outrageous chorus of sucking noises from the guys. She did her best to ignore it. A while later one of the senior community workers got the same treatment when she walked by the group.

(Community centre)

We have already indicated how strange the area and its people sometimes seemed to us as outsiders. It was not that the local people were in any way inhospitable; on the contrary, they were generally very open in their dealings with us. Rather, it had more to do with the lack of shared experience between ourselves and local people. Lacking the bedrock of shared lives we often felt as though we were in an entirely foreign culture in which we were simply at a loss at times to know how to interpret people's statements or behaviour.

In one-to-one contact with local people it was not difficult to tap into the enormous and continuing sadness of family lives that had been undermined in some way as a result of widespread drug use:

I sat drinking coffee with Mary in the canteen area. I asked her if she ever got worried that her son would take to drugs. 'Eh, I've got two sons, both of them junkies.' At this point Mary's daughter came over and asked what we were talking about. The daughter then said that her mother had had a terrible time of it, always stealing stuff off her. 'They've taken everything. It's worst at Christmas when you've all the presents in.' Mary then talked about how she had to walk around at home 'with her purse up her arse' as if that were the only safe place to leave it. She described a situation where she'd been 'away to make the tea' and had to stop it mid-way because she had forgotten her purse. 'I went and got it and the two of them were looking at me and I said "what are you lookin' at it's cos of you two I have to keep ma purse with me" . . .' Mary seemed to display a mixture of anger, disgust and hopelessness when she spoke of her sons. Her daughter though was less conciliatory, she felt that they ought to have been put out of the house.

(Community centre)

The great majority of the people we contacted had personal experience of others who injected drugs. It was common to find that even if the person we were talking to did not inject drugs he or she had a brother or sister who did:

'All my brother's friends and the ones I know, the mature ones, I mean they have been junkies longer than the ones I went to school with. I see them, I know them, I know of them, 30 or 40 names that I could say that's Peter, that's Paul, or that's Mary, that's Jeannie or Peter's sister or that's somebody you know. I know who people are . . . there's always somebody that knows someone very well that's on drugs. There is always a relation or very close friend. Everybody knows about it.'

(Community centre)

Drug use as distinct from drug injecting seemed to have become an almost mundane feature of everyday life in the area. Many young adolescents reported smoking cigarettes and cannabis, experimenting with alcohol and tablets, as well as inhalants like glue:

Lynn who's 13 described a hideout she'd made in a basement of a derelict tenement. 'We done it up, put a carpet in, some car seats, music and smoked hash.' I asked her about smoking hash she replied, 'oh aye, I've been smoking it for a good while now, everyone's into it.'

(IT)

Sally (13) made frequent reference to the amount of glue she's been sniffing lately. She also said she'd been smoking cannabis and had also swallowed temazepam. I asked how she'd got hold of these things, 'ma dad deals it, I stole it off him.'

(IT)

Many young people were using drugs recreationally, for instance on a night out with friends at a disco:

We were walking down the main street when we met Eddie, a non-injector. He was eager to tell us of his recent experiences with Ecstacy in one of the town clubs. 'You know, there's nae cunt that would've talked me into tryin' anything like that. I've never used any drugs but when I went down there and saw them all dancin', I thought I'm gonnae try some of that.'

(Streetwork field-note)

Many of the drugs that were being used were also potentially addictive. We noticed, however, that although drugs were categorized in terms of their addictiveness, the criteria for doing so had less to do with the pharmacological properties of the drug than the kinds of situation they were used in, the means of taking them and the type of person taking them. This seemed the case from the schoolchildren's response to our query as to whether or not people could take drugs in a controlled manner and avoid addiction:

'Aye, but it depends on the person, you could be taking a lot of different drugs but that wouldn't necessarily mean you were a junkie.' Another added 'there are people who take sulph. and that, but they're no' junkies.'

(School)

A drug which was swallowed and used for a specifically social purpose, like going dancing, was viewed differently from when it was injected:

I asked what drugs they felt it was okay to take. One boy said it was alright to take pills 'there's lots of people do that, for the dancing.' He said he wouldn't try to stop a friend from taking pills, that wasn't perceived by him as worrying, only injecting was, then he would be concerned.

(School)

Although none of the non-injectors we contacted saw themselves as being seriously involved in the use of drugs, the majority of them had direct personal experience of them. Given the widespread availability of drugs this is perhaps not surprising. Drugs are commonplace in this area, and the readiness of many young people we met to experiment with them suggests that at least some will, in time, go on to injecting drug use.

Contacting drug injectors

In a study such as this, one needs lucky breaks either in the contacts that are made or in the information provided. In this study we were fortunate to make contact with a local pharmacist who had begun to sell sterile injecting equipment at low cost as a way of reducing the spread of HIV infection in the area. The pharmacist was happy to work with us and offered part of his shop as a setting where we could interview people who came in to buy needles and syringes. This offer proved invaluable and we were able to interview 102 injectors within this setting alone. In addition, one of us worked in the local needle exchange over an eight-month period during which time we were able to interview 50 people and to develop research relationships with many others. Our presence within the pharmacy and the needle exchange was also invaluable in other less tangible respects. If one's only contact with drug injectors is in a hospital or drug treatment setting there is a tendency to view drug use, either implicitly or explicitly, as a deviant practice. Part of the reason for this has to do with the fact that within such settings one tends to see only individuals whose drug use has begun to cause problems. What one misses are those individuals for whom drug injecting is only one, and by no means necessarily the most important, aspect of their lives.

Spending time within the pharmacy and the needle exchange enabled us to contact a spectrum of individuals from those who could be considered as 'addicts' to those who were injecting only on an occasional basis and whose drug injecting had not, as yet at least, become problematic. Interviewing people within these settings was also valuable in enabling us to build up contacts with local injectors and to gain access to their informal gatherings on the streets. As with each aspect of our work it was necessary to progress with caution so as not to engender suspicions amongst local drug injectors as to our motives:

> In the pharmacy today Pat (injector) mentioned having seen Neil at the intersection of two streets where drug injectors often congregate. 'He was reading a paper. I didnae go up to him, you know he's a stranger, people don't know his face. He could be the polis or some-thing. I know he's not but they might not. I made eye contact but I didnae talk to him. If I had, people would have wanted to know who he was and all. It would have been like the French Inquisition.' The pharmacist said to Pat that if he saw any heavy men with Neil he should go over and say he was alright. Pat agreed 'Aye I know he's brand new, I know the guy and what he does but he's still a stranger.'
>
> (Pharmacy)

Gradually, however, our contacts with local drug injectors acquired an easygoing familiarity that enabled us to extend our work onto the streets:

This afternoon I decided to spend time standing by the railings near the pharmacy – something which I notice many drug injectors do. After 15 or so minutes someone approached me from behind, put something at my back, and said 'your money or you'll get a doin'. I turned to see Jack's smiling face (I had spoken to him on many previous occasions when he had been in buying needles). We chatted for a good 40 minutes or so about his brother who was due for an operation, about a recent drugs raid on his family's flat and about his own forthcoming trial. As we chatted various other drug users came over and offered Jack advice, what to say to his lawyer, the judge, etc. What was good about this contact was that I didn't feel at all ill at ease.

(Streetwork field-note)

Over time these contacts extended to the hinterland of streets behind the pharmacy where many of the drug injectors lived and where they would inject in some of the semi-derelict boarded up tenements.

This developing familiarity meant that we were able to spend many evenings walking around the estate and standing chatting with small group-ings of drug injectors. Over time we became, it seemed, a relatively ac-cepted part of the street scene:

Whilst we were sitting with Robby a young guy came along with his girlfriend and their dog. The girl asked Robby if he knew who had any Tems. Robby mentioned that someone was away to get some and they were waiting for his return. He came back not long afterwards and the two went with him into the back close where the drugs were dealt. Another girl came along and asked if anyone had jellies. I was surprised that all of this went on without reference to Neil and I. I had thought we might compromise the situation a bit, but this wasn't the case – perhaps because we were in the company of Robby.

(Streetwork field-note)

Despite the familiarity which developed between us and many of the people we were in contact with, there was always a degree to which they managed their interaction with us and sought to put limits on the kinds of information we were privy to:

Neil asked Tomo about the stairwells in two derelict tenement build-ings which we knew were used for the purposes of injecting drugs. Tomo immediately became defensive saying that nobody hit up in there and in fact nobody even went in there. This last assertion was somewhat weakened by the exit of a man during the time we stood with Tomo. Furthermore the stairwell had recently been graffitied and bore the names of many injectors known to us, including Tomo's. It was clear that Tomo not only didn't want to pursue the subject but also that he wanted to dissuade us from going there, his final comment being, 'youse are better off standing out here where people can find you.'

(Streetwork field-note)

At the same time, however, we were able to develop sufficient trust with certain individuals to be given access to their domestic world. At the outset of the study we had assumed, perhaps rather naively, that we would mundanely witness many first-hand instances of needle and syringe sharing. In the main, however, drug injectors often seemed reluctant to inject in front of non-injectors:

> Marina and I walked up into the estate and met up with William – he asked if we wanted to come round to his ma's flat for tea. When we got to the flat a woman was standing outside – she and William chatted together and then we all went up to the flat. The place was really well cared for (William explained that his ma was away). William immediately put the TV on and then left the room. The woman explained that he was off looking for Temgesics. William returned later and asked if we wouldn't mind him having a hit. By this time the woman was already getting the needle/syringe out. She cracked the tablet in two and placed both halves in the syringe barrel and added water and shook the mixture up. I thought she was about to hit up but both she and William went to the kitchen to do this. She reappeared a few moments later carrying a large bowl of water. She sat down and soaked her feet explaining that she had been in the town all day shoplifting.

(Streetwork field-note)

Nevertheless, during the course of our research we were able to directly observe many occasions when injecting equipment was passed between drug injectors even if we were not always able to observe its shared use.

In each of the chapters that follow we draw on data from these different sources to look at various aspects of drug injectors' HIV-related risk behaviour. In this chapter, by contrast, we have tried to convey something of what life was like more generally in the area and have tried to combine this with a portrayal of our work as participant observers in that area.

Chapter 3

Needle and syringe
sharing

Introduction

In the mid-1980s an aspect of drug injectors' behaviour that had excited
little previous interest suddenly became the focus of almost worldwide
concern. The sharing of needles and syringes had been identified as one of
the highest risk practices in the spread of HIV infection, and from that
point on would never again enjoy the relative obscurity of the pre-AIDS
era. Apart from the early classic study conducted in the 1970s by Howard
and Borges (1970), hardly anything was known about the reasons why drug
injectors shared, the situations in which they shared, how often they shared
or with whom they shared. Initial research efforts concentrated on the
frequency with which people shared and the numbers of people involved
(Robertson et al. 1986; Chaisson et al. 1987; Lange, et al. 1987). Although
this information was crucial in estimating the risks of epidemic spread of
HIV infection, detailed information still needed to be collected on the
social dynamics of sharing, its meaning for those individuals involved, and
the way in which it was influenced by local drug using cultures (Des Jarlais
et al. 1986). Information of this kind is crucial not simply in terms of
understanding drug injectors' behaviour, but in devising relevant interventions which might successfully change drug injectors' behaviour and reduce
their risks of contracting and spreading HIV infection.

In looking at AIDS-related risk behaviour there is a danger of concentrating so much on specific risk practices that one ignores the social
context in which behaviour occurs. As Friedman and his colleagues have
recently pointed out:

There is a common conception that the human immunodeficiency
virus (HIV) is transmitted through risky behaviour, and thus that

AIDS among intravenous (IV) drug users is an issue of behaviour and behaviour change. This view is an advance over naive views of risk groups, but is not fully adequate. It needs to be supplemented by a social approach that sees risk as a pattern of interaction in which the virus is transmitted from an infected person to an uninfected person. Such inter-action typically occurs within the framework of, and indeed embodies, a social relationship.

(Friedman *et al.* 1990a: 85)

We would go further than this in suggesting that drug injectors' risk behaviour needs to be understood not only in terms of the social relationships between drug injectors, but also in terms of the local culture shared between people generally living within an area. Before looking in detail at the sharing of injecting equipment, we will therefore consider more broadly sharing between people living in the area where many of our contacts with drug injectors were established.

Sharing and the wider social environment

Although one of the most noticeable features of the area was the level of deterioration of the physical surroundings there was also a highly developed sense of neighbourliness and mutual support amongst people generally:

This evening I had arranged to go and hear one of the local voluntary workers playing in his band in the local pub. When I arrived someone called out my name and I recognised one of the lads from the community centre. Chippy (the guy from the band) beckoned me over to a table where he was sat with a group of others. He explained that they would be back on in a few minutes. Chippy introduced me to the others and one of the guys asked me if I wanted a drink. I explained that I only had a small amount of money and that I could not afford to buy a round so thanks but no thanks. In reply he simply asked again if I wanted a drink so I said I would have a half of lager. I immediately regretted this since I noticed that all the other men had pints. While he was away getting my drink one of the women leaned over and said that her man could come down to the pub with only a few bob and come home drunk, 'people will buy for him all evening and when he has money he'll do the same for them.' At this point it occurred to me how nonsensical in their terms my earlier reply had been.

(Streetwork field-note)

This field extract instances only one of numerous occasions when resources were shared as a matter of course between local people. The degree to which seemingly anything and everything was shared between people was striking, particularly given the level of widespread deprivation which characterized the area.

As well as being commonplace between people generally in the local area, sharing was also widespread amongst the drug injectors:

> We went back into the sitting room where Clare shared out the last of her cigarettes – 'See it's funny there's a lot of straight people who keep their fags to themselves, saying they only smoke their own, but I can't be bothered with that. Most junkies are awful kind-hearted, well generous with their fags.'
>
> (Residential drug detoxification unit)

In terms of a concern with HIV spread it obviously makes sense to distinguish between the sharing of injecting equipment, and the sharing of such everyday items as food, clothing, alcohol and cigarettes. The point, however, is that the sharing of needles and syringes between drug injectors may be part of a broader culture of neighbourliness and mutual support between people generally living within an area:

> Jimmy showed us into his flat and immediately began preparing his hit. He got some water and put it into the syringe, added the Tems and began shaking them until they dissolved. When they dissolved he stuck the spike on and put a rope around his arm. Then he stuck his arm, drew the blood back into the barrel before withdrawing the needle and cleaning his arm with a swab. Jimmy had just finished hitting up when someone rang from downstairs asking if he would let them in so they could hit up in the close. Jimmy let them into the close but said he did not let anyone hit up in his flat. 'It'd be a mess, there'd be people cleaning their works all over the carpet. No I give them water and they can hit up in the close.' The door-bell rang and it was someone wanting to know if Jimmy wanted to buy some blue socks. Then again someone came to the door and asked if Jimmy could lend a set of tools out. He came in and got a spare set out. I asked if that happened a lot, 'Aye, maybe 5 times a day. I don't like to see anyone strung out so I give them a set if I have one. I'd not give them a brand new set though.' The person at the door seemed to want to come in but Jimmy knocked her/him back saying 'I've got company . . . They'll not bother me if I say I've got company.'
>
> (Streetwork field-note)

This extract is particularly interesting since it well illustrates a level of neighbourliness often held to be a traditional aspect of close knit working class communities. It is not difficult to see how such reciprocity might in part explain the sharing of injecting equipment in those inner city working class communities throughout Britain where drug use has become increasingly prevalent in the last ten years (Pearson 1987; Parker *et al.* 1988).

Recent ethnographic work from Amsterdam and also San Francisco similarly makes the point that sharing behaviour has a broader social context than the sharing of needles and syringes (Feldman and Biernacki 1988; Grund *et al.* 1991).

Stressing the importance of a wider culture of mutual support and neighbourliness only highlights a single aspect of the local culture which might falsely present a rather romanticized view of relationships. As we will show at a later point in the chapter, peer intimidation between drug injectors also influenced the sharing of injecting equipment.

In the next section, however, we look at the social organization of syringe sharing, and examine the distinction between lending and borrowing injecting equipment as well as the way in which these activities were influenced by the social relationships between drug injectors.

The social organization of syringe sharing

The popular image of drug users sharing each others' injecting equipment consists of a large group of people chaotically passing around a single needle and syringe whilst experiencing the effects of a drug-induced stupor. Although this scenario might hold on a few occasions, in fact the sharing of injecting equipment was a more socially patterned activity than this suggests. Drug injectors themselves often rejected this representation of their behaviour:

> Sandra commented on an advert she had seen on television to discourage people from taking drugs describing it as a room full of people hitting up and indiscriminately using dirty needles from ashtrays 'junkies are not manky like that, those adverts are not real, I've never seen anyone do that.'
>
> (Needle exchange)

One aspect of the sharing of injecting equipment which such an image misses entirely is the distinction between lending and borrowing. This distinction is important partly because the two activities differ markedly in their personal risk of HIV and in their risk of generating epidemic spread of HIV infection (McKeganey *et al.* 1989). It is also important because it clearly illustrates that sharing is not generally a random activity, but a highly selective one which belies popular stereotypes of drug injectors.

Lending and borrowing

Borrowing someone else's previously used needles and syringes is an activity which carries a high personal risk for the borrower. In terms of generating epidemic spread of HIV infection, however, such borrowing is a relatively low risk activity. So long as the person lending the equipment does not re-use it then it is only the borrower who risks becoming infected. On the other hand, lending is an activity that carries little personal risk (so long as the lender does not re-use the equipment), but is of high risk in terms of epidemic spread of HIV. The lender can, at no risk to him or herself, generate an epidemic of infection amongst all of those to whom needles and syringes have been passed.

This distinction is also important because drug injectors themselves often made reference to borrowing or lending (using either these or equivalent terms) in describing their own activities. A sizeable minority of the people we have spoken to, for example, described themselves as neither lending nor borrowing injecting equipment:

> I asked Helen when she had last shared. She thought back and said 'about two years ago now. I don't share with anyone, not even my brothers.' I asked if she got asked to lend her works. 'No, I'll not lend them to anyone. I don't get asked. They know I'll not lend them, that's why. Even my brother, he asked for a lend and I says no. He says "why, how come, you think I've got the virus or something?" I say "No, Tim, you'll have to get your own, I'll not lend them." '
>
> (Pharmacy)

This attitude is quite encouraging in terms of HIV-related risk reduction. However, it was much more common for people to say that although they themselves would not use other people's injecting equipment they would pass on their own equipment if asked to do so. Over 80 people said that they had, and would, pass on their equipment in this way, adding that they would not then re-use it:

> 'I wouldnae use other people's but if somebody wanted mine I would give them a used set but I wouldnae use them again.'
>
> (Pharmacy)

> 'I don't use anyone else's works, not even my girlfriend's who also hits up. That's why I buy two sets, one for her and one for me. There's people that come up and say "Can I have a lend of your tools?" and I just give them ones I've used and say "Do what you like with them and throw them away." '
>
> (Needle exchange)

In contrast to people who said they would lend, but not borrow, a few people described themselves as both lending and borrowing:

I asked Ian when he had last shared. He laughed at this and said 'Yesterday. When you're choking for a hit and you've not got works you'll use anyone's.' It was Sunday. In response to my question would he share with someone who was HIV positive he said 'Well, I'd try not to be in a situation where I'd share with one of them.' I said 'but what if you were choking?' He laughed and said 'You would use it if it were a nail with a hole in it so you would when you're choking. Everyone shares, even though they say no. Aye, they're kidologists, especially in . . . where it's difficult to get works'. I asked him if he'd lend his works out. 'Depends on how many other sets I've got.'

(Needle exchange)

I asked Pete whether he had shared much – 'All the time. I've used every cunt's needles, even people that have got the virus. I haven't shared since I came out of jail in January. I got the results of my test. It was negative. I went up the same time as Simon. We got our results at the same time.' I asked about sharing in jail – 'Oh aye, usually there will be about 10 all sitting round and they'll use the one set.' He then said he'd been sharing his sister's needles between two to five times a week. 'Aye, but she's had the test and she's negative so I'm alright aren't I?'

(Needle exchange)

Although the drug injector in the extract above freely described himself as sharing 'all the time' such people were often described by others in negative terms:

I asked if people often asked for a lend of her works. She replied 'well, there's that . . . he often comes up to me and to . . . and asks for a lend of my tools. He never buys them although if you're getting enough for a score deal I can't see how you can't afford a set of tools. I mean 39p, that's not much is it? I say to him "You're going to have to start getting yourself your own sets", but he says "well, it's alright from you and . . . because I know you don't share, I only get them from you people because you're alright."'

(Hospital detoxification unit)

I asked Freddie if people asked to use his tools and he interpreted this to mean whether he was sharing himself – 'No I'm in the chemist four times a day getting my needles'. I repeated my question about other people and he said 'Oh there's that manky bastard Mickey he's always asking – I cannae tell you how many times he's round my house saying "Gonnae give me a lend of your works?"'

(Streetwork field-note)

Only very few people described themselves as borrowing, but not lending. On the whole this tended to occur where the sharing itself was seen as part of a particular relationship, rather than as something which could be extended to include others:

> I asked Sharon if she worried about sharing needles. She said 'I only share with my best pal. We mix around. Sometimes she uses mine, sometimes I use hers. Maybe it's difficult for you to understand if you aren't a junkie but maybe one day she'll say "First hit's mine" and next day I'll say "First hit's mine" – like that, all mixed around.' She said she didn't lend out her works – 'Sometimes I'll just be sitting down to my tea and the door will go. Someone will be there saying "Can I have a lend of your works?" I just say "I've not got works to lend because I don't want to get into that."'
>
> (Hospital detoxification unit)

So far in this section we have outlined the range of responses to lending and borrowing amongst the drug injectors. In qualitative studies such as ours it is often not possible to quantify people's responses in relation to specific behaviour patterns. Nevertheless, in the retail pharmacy we did employ a limited set of questions which were asked of most of the drug injectors interviewed in that setting. In Table 1 we have summarized the information on lending and borrowing to give some idea of the frequency of these behaviours.

Table 1 Needle and syringe sharing

	Male (n = 74)	Female (n = 23)	Total (n = 97)
Report being asked to pass on used needles and syringes	43 (58.1%)	15 (65.2%)	58 (59.8%)
Report having recently used others' previously used injecting equipment	20 (27.0%)	4 (17.4%)	24 (24.7%)
Report having recently passed on or being prepared to pass on injecting equipment	40 (54.1%)	15 (65.2%)	55 (56.7%)
Report being prepared neither to pass on nor to use another's injecting equipment	23 (31.1%)	5 (21.7%)	28 (28.8%)

Social relationships of sharing

What is striking from the accounts of those lending and those borrowing injecting equipment is the degree to which the assessment of one's personal relationship with the individual concerned impinges upon the decision to share. This has similarly been found in a recent study of injectors in Seattle in the United States (Calsyn *et al.* 1991). It is evident that for many of the drug injectors social distance had a direct bearing on decisions to share injecting equipment. Most of the sharing that we have identified, for example, was between sexual partners:

> She had a boyfriend whom she finished with in January. He was using drugs as well and they shared works. She said she wasn't worried about catching the virus from him because he would only use his own works.
>
> (Hospital detoxification ward)

Similarly,

> I asked Irene about hitting up and sharing equipment and she said she only used her boyfriend's tools – 'We'd go in and buy one set.' Asked if she had not been worried about AIDS to the degree of buying her own tools she said 'No, you don't think about that when you're wanting a hit', then she noted it was only her boyfriend whom she had shared with – 'Aye, but don't get me wrong. These people come up to the door for a loan of works and I give them an old set and say they can keep them.'
>
> (Needle exchange)

Sharing with one's sexual partner was described more often by women than men. This may be largely due to the fact, as we will show in Chapter 5, that the majority of female drug injectors were in relationships with drug injecting males whereas only a minority of males had drug injecting female partners. However, by no means all drug injectors living together shared each other's injecting equipment. Some people would go to quite extraordinary lengths to avoid using their partner's needles and syringes:

> In response to my question about sharing needles she answered, 'Never, see like just now, I stayed with a lassie and a guy and we all have a wee box each with our names written on it and when we take a hit we put our works back in the wee poke and we don't get them mixed up that way. I've been asked to lend them out right enough but I just say "that's you then but I don't want them back".'
>
> (Pharmacy)

Minimizing the risk of sharing in this way was mentioned by only a small number of people.

In addition to sharing between sexual partners a few people reported sharing with other family members, most often with siblings, but as the following example shows, not necessarily only them:

> 'Couple of nights back I used a needle that had been used by my two

cousins because I was choking. If someone was rattlin' I'd give them a set but I'd not take them back.'

(Pharmacy)

Sharing was also widely described as occurring between 'best friends':

I asked about needle sharing – 'I only use his (pointing to his friend) and he doesnae use anybody elses. We don't share all the time, no, we usually have our own sets but if we don't then we'll just use each other's.' I had the odd sensation of talking to one person in two bodies when I talked to these lads.

(Needle exchange)

It is interesting that some people did not consider sharing with their best friend or partner as sharing at all; sharing for them involved passing one's injecting equipment on to other people who were more distant.

This group of 3 men said that they got asked for needles by others 'but we dinnae let other people have them.' They also said that they shared amongst themselves. When I asked if they were not worried about one of them having/getting AIDS one said 'I'm just out of jail and they took my blood there. They would have told me if I had AIDS so I know I'm in the clear.' I asked if he had been hitting up in jail. 'Yea' and then one of the others said 'I took tools up to him.' The other one then said that he had left his tools behind. If this guy was in a cell with others I'd be really surprised if he had not shared with them if they were also injectors and had drugs to take.

(Pharmacy)

Sharing in large groups was more frequently mentioned by men than women, although it did not appear to be a common occurrence for either. On the few occasions of group sharing that were reported it was clear that there was considerable potential for infection to occur:

I asked Phil if he'd shared in the last three months. 'Aye, well I'll be full of it and the table will be just full of works, you'll come out of a gouch like and take the nearest ones to you and say to yourself they look like mine but how d'ye know? They might be anybody's and then you just use them.'

(Needle exchange)

There were also reports of one or two individuals who allowed others to inject in their home in exchange for small quantities of drugs. On such occasions use would sometimes be made of injecting equipment that was already within the house. This created the possibility of serial anonymous sharing occurring between people and has to be seen as a situation of very high risk even though it was not commonly reported.

Perhaps most worrying of all, though, were the frequent reports provided by HIV positive drug injectors of being asked to pass on their needles and syringes to others who actually knew their HIV positive diagnosis:

The boy who was HIV positive said there was still a lot of sharing happening in the area. 'I've had people come up to me and ask for ma works. I tell them I have the virus but they still ask.' The boy with the virus said that he felt that if a junkie had smack and no works he'd always use someone else's rather than go without – 'Like he (his mate) had a set that was blocked so I gave him mine that I hadnae used for months so if anything was in it would be dead.'

(Pharmacy)

Clare said that people have asked her sister Elaine if they could have a lend of her works even though they know she's got the virus. 'Elaine's straight with them. She says "No, I've got the virus" but some persist saying "No, it's O.K. I'll sterilise them with bleach".' Clare herself said that if she's in a situation where she is going to share she'll usually try to give them a clean with Dettol.

(Hospital detoxification ward)

Some of the drug injectors we contacted reported having used the equipment of people whom they knew or suspected to be HIV positive:

'Last night – I used them third, but there were five of us. I don't know how much good it does but I try to clean mine. See, when you clean them in the water and then there's some blood – well, when it comes to ma turn I take the water and I change it again before using it.' He says he's using every day and that he's sharing every day. 'I go next door to my pal but I have to be quick 'cos he might not have any. I mostly use his but I don't just use his. I sometimes share with a guy who I think might have AIDS. I try to clean the tools. I did use bleach once but he saw. I tried to hide it but I dropped it on my sweater and made a hole. I don't think he suspected I was doing it because I think he's got AIDS.'

(Needle exchange)

We talked about drug use, HIV risks and AIDS and Christine said that she shared with lots of people. I asked her when the last time was. 'Last week. I met a boy here and we went shoplifting in B.H.S. We got some stuff, sold it and bought some smack. It was about 4.00 in the afternoon in the south side. I didnae have a set of works and he said "you cannae use mine because I have the virus". I said "dinnae bother, so do I" which I don't but I knew he would not have let me have a hit otherwise. He knows that I have two wee ones and he didnae want to be the one to give me the virus. I don't think I'll get the virus though because I've shared with lots of people and I'm still negative but he only shared a few times and got the virus.' I asked Christine if she felt that everyone who had the virus would die of AIDS. 'I don't know. It's got to do something to you, but I don't know if it would kill you.' I asked her if she was worried about AIDS at all and she shook her head and mumbled 'No.'

(HIV counselling clinic)

We look at the reactions of drug injectors and others to AIDS and HIV infection in Chapter 6. It is important to note that most of the HIV positive drug injectors we spoke to felt able to turn down requests to lend their injecting equipment. A few individuals did, however, feel that their obligation to other injectors extended only to letting the person know of their HIV status, leaving it up to the individual to decide whether or not to make use of the equipment (McKeganey 1990).

So far in this chapter we have described sharing within the context of people's everyday lives. Sharing also occurs, however, within certain institutional settings, most notably within prisons and residential drug detoxification units:

He said that when he'd been in Key West (drug de-tox unit) there had been a boy there with the virus. I asked if the guy had told him that himself. 'Aye, a set of works got brought in and he said "Listen guys, I'd like to use them but I've got the virus so I'll need to go last". I went first.' I asked him if he'd brought the works in. 'Aye, it was me.'

(Needle exchange)

When asked about sharing Tony said 'I'm just out of the jail and I was usin' works there that had gone around thirty people.'

(Pharmacy)

Both prisons and residential drug detoxification units are settings which have resident populations of drug injectors. Both settings place limits on the availability of sterile injecting equipment and both are subject, to an unknown degree, to inmates successfully smuggling drugs and needles on to the premises (Bloor *et al.* 1989). The shared use of unsterile injecting equipment within both of these settings may pose an especially high risk of infection given the limited scope for sterilizing injecting equipment:

Earlier in our conversation Billy had talked about being in prison saying that he had not used at all when inside. 'It's a funny thing but when I'm inside I never use. I smoke hash but I never hit up.' Billy then described how at Grange prison when he had recently been there, of the 25 blokes in his part, at least 12 had been using one set of tools. I asked about cleaning tools and he said you could only rinse them in the sink and that the water was pretty filthy.

(Streetwork field-note)

In the next section we will look in detail at those factors which seemed to influence the sharing of injecting equipment.

The influence of sharing

In reviewing all of the occasions of needle and syringe sharing that were described to us six factors, operating either individually or in concert, appear to be particularly influential. It is important to stress that the six influences we have identified are not mutually exclusive.

1 Accidental or inadvertent sharing
2 Availability of sterile injecting equipment
3 Need to inject
4 Individual assessment of risk
5 Social norms
6 Nature of the relationship involved

Accidental or inadvertent sharing

Although almost all of the sharing so far described could be seen as consciously motivated, some sharing was occurring inadvertently as a result of confusion arising over the ownership of injecting equipment:

> When he came in he said he thought he had Hepatitis adding that he did not know how he could have got it. I asked him if he had ever lent his tools and he said that he had lent out a brand new set and then put them under his bed, so maybe, he added, they got mixed up.
>
> (Needle exchange)

The scope for such accidental or inadvertent sharing was itself influenced by underlying notions of ownership. Some individuals, for example, appeared to maintain a clear sense of personally owning their injecting equipment such that confusion as to who owned which needle was unlikely to occur:

> I then asked Gail about sharing other people's tools. She said that she did not use other people's tools but she did get asked for hers and in such situations would give a set away. 'I scratch my initial on my own set and if I get asked I give them another set.' I asked Gail if it was difficult to say no in such circumstances. 'Aye, if you say no, people ask "why no?" They say they don't have the virus or they think you have the virus.' I then asked Gail if she had been in situations where groups of people had been hitting up and sharing tools, whether it had been difficult to decline sharing. She agreed that yes, it had and that on such occasions she had shared. 'I've been in situations where that's

happened and where there's been people who've been off it and others have said you go and have a hit because they don't like to see people who are off it.'

(HIV counselling clinic)

Other individuals, by contrast, were more lax in their control over their equipment and presumably more likely to accidentally or unknowingly share equipment:

> I asked Steve if he was worried about AIDS/HIV. He said he was and I then asked him about needle sharing. He said that he shared other people's tools and I asked him to describe the last situation where this had occurred. 'Ma mate and I had got kit and we went round this guy's house and used the set of tools that were there. I had previously left my old set of tools there the night before when I was completely out of it. Anyway, this time we got there and there was a set of works sitting in a glass of water which I used.' I asked Steve if he had cleaned the works out and whether there was any antiseptic in the glass. It wasn't that he found the latter amusing, more that it was simply not something he had thought about – 'No, I think it was just water. I used them and ma mate did too and then we left, leaving the tools behind.' At this point I asked Steve why he hadn't purchased a clean set of tools and he said simply that he was in a hurry.

(HIV counselling clinic)

Availability

An important determinant of sharing is the availability of sterile injecting equipment (Power 1988; Stimson *et al.* 1988). Perhaps the clearest example of this is where sharing occurs in those settings where formal constraints are placed on the availability of injecting equipment:

> I asked Gerry to describe the last time he shared. 'It was two months ago. I was in prison and although I had ma own needle ma mother would no' bring me any smack in. There was this guy in the next cell though who had smack shoved up his arse but no needles. I said he could use ma tools if he let me have some of his smack which he did.' I asked Gerry if he had cleaned his tools and he said he had with hot water though not because he was worried about AIDS but in order that they would work alright.

(HIV counselling clinic)

Where injecting drug use occurs within such a setting an individual may find it extremely difficult to resist the demands of others to use his or her injecting equipment.

Whilst some sharing undoubtedly arose as a direct result of sterile injecting equipment not being available in situations where injecting took place, it is also the case that availability itself is partly rooted in drug injectors' behaviour:

> I asked him about sharing, he replied, 'The last few days we've been using each others'.' I asked him and his friend why that was, was it because they did not have enough money to buy clean sets? 'That and also being too lazy to go up the road to get some.'
>
> (Needle exchange)

The extent to which availability of sterile injecting equipment is in part dependent upon the behaviour of individual injectors is further illustrated in the following extract:

> When he first started injecting he wouldn't share his tools/works with anyone – 'For the first 3 weeks or so I wouldn't share but then the shop (chemist) might be closed because it's late and so you share once and then after that you think "Oh fuck it" and take the risk. Any junkie who tells you that he's never shared needles is a liar.' He described the last time he had shared works with anyone which was about 3 weeks ago. He was with a girl and boy. 'I'm not going to mention their names'. They're not people Simon usually 'jumps about with'. They went to a pub in a neighbouring area where they could buy Tems. They had enough money for a taxi there but had to walk back. Knowing this and not wanting to walk back 'without being full of it' they planned it by taking a bottle of water so as they could inject themselves. On the golf course they all sat down and took their hits. Neil asked if there weren't other people there. Simon laughed 'Oh yes, but we didn't care.' At this point I questioned Simon about this incident in the light of his aforementioned worry about HIV. I asked him if they'd planned it so much as to get the water, didn't they think to buy needles also? He shrugged at this – 'No, we just took the one set.'
>
> (Hospital detoxification unit)

The group had planned their expedition to the extent that they carried water with them for dissolving the tablets to inject them, but this did not extend to ensuring an adequate supply of clean needles and syringes. Other individuals, by contrast, planned ahead so as to avoid the possibility of having to share:

> He asked what the research was about and as soon as I mentioned needle sharing said 'Oh, I don't do any of that'. He says the last time he shared was about 3 years ago (1985). 'Just about the time the AIDS thing got started'. He was motivated then by a worry of Hepatitis. There was apparently a lot of it about and so he started to buy his own

needles and wouldn't share. He says he cannot remember a time when he's been caught short. On a Saturday he buys one set which he uses 2/3 times and then flings it away down the stank.

(Hospital detoxification unit)

Need to inject

In a situation where sterile injecting equipment was unavailable an individual might seek to avoid sharing by postponing his or her drug use:

'I don't share though there's people that have asked for a loan of ma works. If the chemist was shut I wouldn't share. I just wouldn't bother having a hit.'

(Pharmacy)

More common than the preparedness to postpone or cease injecting was the feeling that in a situation where drugs were available, but sterile injecting equipment was not, most people would ignore the risks and share:

Mark confirmed Neil's question as to whether or not he got worse withdrawals when he had the drugs in his hand. 'See, sometimes I've left ma tools at home and I'm off, running like a greased bullet.' The worst though was when someone had gone off into town to get Tems (say 20–30) and everyone would be waiting and waiting for the person to return. – 'When he got off the bus they'd be there like a swarm. If you're in that situation and you don't have spare works then you share. It always happens like that.'

(Hospital detoxification unit)

As an alternative to sharing one could, of course, choose to swallow, smoke or snort one's drugs:

'I don't share ma works with anybody – see I've been where I've had no works of ma own and I've asked Eileen and she's said "I've only got these but they're used, you can have them if you want" but I've said "nothing against you Eileen but I'd rather crush it (the tablet) down and snort it" and that's what I've done in front of her and snorted it. "Nothing wrong with you Eileen – I wouldnae use them after ma Granny or anybody".'

(Needle exchange)

In practice, however, only very few people seemed prepared to consider such an option. This is illustrated in Table 2 which summarizes our data from the retail pharmacy.

Table 2 Prepared to switch from injecting to snorting

	Males (n = 69)	Females (n = 18)	Total (n = 87)
Would make change	5 (7.2%)	2 (11.1%)	7 (8.0%)
Would not make change	62 (89.9%)	16 (88.9%)	78 (89.6%)
Don't know	2 (2.9%)	—	2 (2.2%)

Individual assessment of risk

For many of the drug injectors the decision to share injecting equipment was influenced in part by their assessment of the likely risks involved. Selecting an individual who was regarded as 'clean' was described as one way of reducing the risks of sharing:

> Earlier I'd asked Peter if he used other people's works. 'There is no need. The chemist is just up the road.' I said I'd heard there was more sharing going on now – 'That's a load of shite, absolute shite.' I said 'but there must be times when you've been stuck for a needle?' – 'Aye, there's been times when I've been desperate, later in the evening, something like that, but even then I try to be careful who I choose.' Marina – 'what, someone who looks healthy?' – 'Yes, someone who I know doesn't share their works with people.' Helen added that she always used her own spikes but she did give them away when she'd finished if someone wanted them – 'But that's it. I don't take them back.'
>
> (Residential detoxification unit)

Just as sharing itself seemed to be influenced by notions of social distance, so too were the judgements about who was 'clean' and who was 'dirty'. Family members or close friends were often cited as examples of people who were believed to be clean:

> Jim talked about being in a situation of having to borrow someone else's works saying that he had used the tools of one of his two brothers. He added 'they're alright, they're clean.' I asked him how he decided if someone was alright. He laughed 'I don't know, I suppose it's just that I know them.'
>
> (Streetwork field-note)

Similarly, people who were described as dirty were most often people that the individual did not know well. Judgements of not being clean were also focused on fellow drug injectors who were HIV positive, as well as the family members of HIV positive drug injectors:

I asked Sally when the last time she had shared needles was and she said she couldn't remember but didn't think it was long ago. 'I've been with people who wanted to use ma works and I say it's O.K. I'm clean, I've no got anything'. Some do use her tools she said but others say that they will go along to the chemist. Sally added, 'I think it's because ma sister's got the virus and they think I must have it too.'

(Hospital detoxification unit)

Judgements as to how 'clean' or 'dirty' an individual was were also based on an assessment of how discriminating the person was in terms of who he or she shared with:

She described the last time she shared needles as bein, one month ago – 'Aye, about a month ago. I was at my pal's and my spike blocked and rather than running down to the chemist and losin' my hit I borrowed her spike . . . Did I mind? Aye, I minded because she's not fussy about who borrows her works.' She described being really worried because of AIDS saying she was afraid of getting it.

(Drug detoxification unit)

Similar assessments were also made on the basis of whether the person had shared in the past with a particular individual without experiencing any health problems:

I asked Timmy who came in today with a prescription whether he felt needles should be made available at night. He said that he wondered if it was necessary since anyone who wanted them could get them during the day. However, I then asked if people asked for a loan of his tools at night. 'Oh aye, last Sunday I was with a guy who had left his tools in his house and he wanted a shot of mine. I said he should go down and get his own but he said "Look, I've used yours before and I'm okay so I'll just use them the now". I said "Go ahead and keep them because there was no way I was gonnae use them again".'

(Pharmacy)

Minimizing the risks of sharing in this way though was by no means equally pressing for all drug injectors. Some individuals articulated a belief that they perhaps had a 'natural' immunity from infection:

'See I think I'm immune to that AIDS. I've been batterin' my veins now for 13 years and I've had hep twice. That's why I think I'm immune to it. It's like I said, I've never seen anyone who's had hep who's now got AIDS. I think you get immune if you've had hep.'

(Needle exchange)

Others seemed to have adopted a rather fatalistic attitude towards HIV infection:

> I talked about AIDS/HIV to which Joe replied 'If it's for you it'll no' go past you,' adding that he wasn't worried about AIDS at all. A bit surprised by Joe's answer I asked if that meant that he had not changed his drug use since AIDS/HIV. 'No' he replied. Asked directly about sharing he said 'if you want a hit and it's there and you've no' got your own works you'll use somebody elses.' Asked if he meant that he himself would share, he agreed that yes, he would, and he had.
>
> (Residential detoxification unit)

Finally, at least some drug injectors seemed prepared to share others' injecting equipment with little or no regard for the risks involved. Perhaps the clearest indication of this could be seen on those occasions when people reported that they would be prepared to use the equipment of someone who was known to be HIV positive.

Social norms

At the outset we noted how widespread sharing was between local people and how this extended to virtually every aspect of their everyday lives. Since many drug injectors had friends who also injected it is hardly surprising that responses to requests to share injecting equipment were often framed in terms of the reciprocal rights and obligations of friendship:

> He said he hadn't shared in a good while. 'I've never been one for sharing, not since I started. See my pals are all clean. Even when I've shared in the past year I've always bleached my works.' I asked about lending. 'Aye my pals ask me sometimes if they havenae got any works. I give them then. I couldnae knock them back because I know they'd not refuse me.'
>
> (Needle exchange)

As well as being influenced by wider social norms to help friends out, it was also clear that many of the drug injectors, having experienced the effects of drug withdrawal themselves, could not then turn down a fellow drug injector in need:

> I asked Tom about the sharing of works and he explained 'I would share even now – you see, if somebody needed works and they couldn't get a clean set they would use what was around and if somebody asked me I would lend them because the situation might be the opposite next time and it might be me that needed them. If you want a hit and haven't got the works you can't say "keep it till the chemist opens up in the morning".'
>
> (Residential detoxification unit)

Turning down a request to share injecting equipment in a situation where importance was placed on the obligations of friendship, was understandably difficult for many people:

I asked him quite a lot about needle sharing, asking if he was in situations where sharing went on. 'Oh aye, I've been in a lot of situations where there's been sharing, lots. In fact I'll give you an example. On Wednesday I went up from my house with five others but I'd forgotten the spike. I had an orange set. Anyway they sat and took their hit with two 2 ml sets because we had 4 eggs (temazepam) each and you can only hit 2 eggs in the 1 mls. They shared these sets and handed them to me but I said "No, I'll be alright".' I asked if he'd had any reaction. 'Aye, one of my pals said "You think there's something wrong with me? You've known me all my life." I said no I didnae think that but I felt I wanted to be careful. I said it's only 'cos of my son, he's all I've got, I've got to be careful.'

(Needle exchange)

However, by no means all of the drug injectors reported experiencing any difficulty in turning down such requests:

I asked Peter if people would ask him for a loan of his works. 'Yes, they ask but I never let them. I tell them that I've had to come up here and if they want tools that's what they have to do.' I asked if they minded him taking such a strong line. 'Some people do but I don't care. When I'm finished with them I throw them away.'

(Needle exchange)

Nature of the relationship involved

We have already shown how the issue of sharing was inextricably linked to the larger issue of the nature of the relationship between drug injectors. As was pointed out earlier, most of the sharing we identified was between sexual partners, close friends and family members; sharing injecting equipment was an integral feature of these relationships. Assessments of the likely risk of sharing, along with judgements as to how 'clean' or 'dirty' the individual was, were also influenced by notions of social distance. Many individuals articulated a belief that by limiting their sharing to their sexual partner they would somehow reduce the risk of infection:

I asked Sally if she had not been worried about sharing needles – 'I thought it would be alright if I kept to ma boyfriend. I don't share with anyone else though there's people that ask in Townlee. There's a lot of sharing 'cos people there don't really care about the virus.'

(HIV counselling clinic)

However, the fragility of this notion of trust between partners is indicated in our data, as well as that of Mulleady and Sherr (1989), by the possibility that at least one of them might share outside of the relationship:

> She says her boyfriend is using in the prison 'I know that he's sharing. He says he doesnae share but ma brothers are in the same wing and they tell me he doesn't care whose tools he uses.'
>
> (Pharmacy)

Amongst those who were just sharing with their sexual partner, a feeling was sometimes expressed that any illness their partner got they also expected to experience:

> 'I've never shared with anyone. Well aye, I've shared with my husband – what he's got I'll get – I know him, he'll no' share outside.'
>
> (Pharmacy)

> 'The way I see it he'll (her husband) get what I get and vice versa. We use each other's needles but we'll not share outside though.'
>
> (Residential detoxification unit)

There is ample evidence in our work of the way in which close bonds between drug injectors influenced their behaviour with each other, including their preparedness to share. Nonetheless, it would be a mistake to assume that all relationships between drug injectors were of this mutually supportive kind:

> I asked him if people got slashed on their faces for punishment (I had noticed that many of the drug injectors we were seeing had been slashed across their faces). He grinned and pulled back his fringe to show me a scar wound. He said 'there's all sorts of reasons, like there's that Phil in Mayfield, he's famous for slashing people who refuse to hand over things he's asked for. Aye, mostly its a punishment for not paying, or if someone's been ripping a guy off he might get slashed.' He said that recently there had been a few guys slashed in the area for selling crushed up slimming pills as heroin.
>
> (Needle exchange)

While we have very little detailed information on the existence of hierarchies between drug injectors, their existence was demonstrated on various occasions. Individuals who were seen as good fighters, as ruthless or capable of mobilizing others to fight on their behalf were often spoken of in a way which indicated respect and caution by other drug injectors:

> We stood at the entrance to one of the pubs adjacent to an area where dealing takes place. The conversation turned to Keith (a guy I had seen the previous night) I asked Harry (drug injector) if Keith was a 'heavy', he replied that he used to be but not now 'He can call a gang

together in no time though, but he seems to think that it's just the same as when he went inside for four years. He seems to forget that the little boys are all big now.' Harry added that he had been really glad when Keith had been sentenced and that he wished that on the previous night (when I'd noticed Keith being quite aggressive towards Harry) that he had told him 'to get to fuck' and leave him alone.

(Streetwork field-note)

It seems highly likely that the place an individual occupies within such a hierarchy might itself influence the likelihood of either being able to decline a request to share or of having ones own request granted. Certainly, there were numerous reports of sharing in prison being influenced by intimidation:

'The last time I shared was in March in Grange prison and I caught hep. I had ma own tools but somebody wanted a loan of them. If I hadnae given them they'd have taken them off me.'

(Pharmacy)

There seems little reason to suppose that such intimidation is limited only to the prison setting.

So far in this chapter we have described selected aspects of the social organization of needle and syringe sharing. We have looked at the division between lending and borrowing and the ways in which these activities were influenced by the nature of the relationships involved. We have also identified six factors which bear directly on needle and syringe sharing. What has been lacking so far, however, is a theoretical framework that will allow us to identify how these six factors might be combined to produce sharing. In the next section we will look at a number of possible explanatory models.

Explaining sharing

That sharing was occurring at all, given the widespread media coverage stressing the risks of HIV infection, may be seen as both regrettable and surprising. In considering why sharing continued to occur a number of possible explanations can be immediately discounted. First, it may be that drug injectors were unaware of the risks involved and were sharing each other's injecting equipment without realizing these dangers. It is relatively easy to discount this explanation given that so many people were passing on their equipment with the stipulation that they did not want it returned. This suggests that they were well aware of the dangers of sharing. Second, it may be thought that drug injectors have little or no concern for their own health and that if they did they would not be injecting drugs in the first place. Again this explanation is easily discounted. That many people were passing on equipment and not accepting its return, or simply refusing to either lend or borrow equipment, indicates a concern for their own health.

A more sophisticated explanation of needle and syringe sharing has been offered by Coleman and Curtis in London (1988) and Robertson and colleagues (1988) in Edinburgh. In essence the suggestion is that although the majority of drug injectors are concerned with minimizing their risks; nevertheless, a small group of injectors are very high risk takers. Coleman and her colleagues, for example, were able to show that the greatest proportion of needle and syringe sharing episodes in their study involved only a small number of injectors. There are two major difficulties with this explanation. First, the model of high and low risk takers is somewhat static in that it does not really give one an indication of the process by which it is decided that sharing will take place. It is not an explanation grounded in the realities of drug injectors' lifestyles. Second, the model does not adequately explain why those individuals who may be classified as low risk takers, nevertheless still share on occasion. This is a major limitation since although the low risk takers might not share very often, they might still be sharing in high risk situations. Therefore, one needs to be able to explain the behaviour of those individuals who share frequently as well as those who share only occasionally.

The principal difficulty with each of these explanations lies in assuming at the outset that sharing needles and syringes is an activity which can be explained either by reference to drug injectors' deviant motivations or to an inadequate knowledge of the risks involved. Instead of looking for an explanation of sharing in terms of the psycho-pathology of individual drug injectors, there is a need to develop a theoretical schema which can explain how the various factors identified as influencing the decision to share may be combined in different ways and in different situations to produce occasional or frequent sharing. The work of Alfred Schutz on the phenomenology of everyday social life is of considerable value in this regard. In using Schutz at this point we are following the suggestion of Michael Bloor who has employed Schutz' work on systems of relevance to analyse aspects of HIV-related risk behaviour (Bloor *et al.* 1991).

Schutz (1970) was interested in identifying and describing the cognitive and perceptual processes underpinning everyday life. According to Schutz an important distinction in terms of people's perception is between those aspects which exist in the background of one's awareness (horizon) and those elements which are at the forefront of one's awareness and which are directly perceived (theme). This distinction is of value in beginning to understand how drug injectors might continue to share injecting equipment despite their knowledge of the risks involved. Whilst drug injectors might be aware of the risks associated with needle and syringe sharing, nevertheless, within any particular situation knowledge of the risks involved will be more or less thematic. A good illustration of this can be seen on those occasions where individuals commented that although they shared injecting equipment with their sexual partner or their best friend they did not perceive this as a risky behaviour.

Within the context of an individual relationship, then, the issue of risk might operate at the level of horizon rather than theme, and not directly impinge on a couple's preparedness to share injecting equipment. It is important to stress, however, that even though the issue of risk might exist at the level of horizon; nevertheless, changes might occur within a relationship that serve to elevate a concern with risk to the level of being thematic:

She says that she and her boyfriend always share the same set of works. She has also shared with him and his sister too, though she added that recently she has been buying two sets of works. I asked her why? 'I don't know. I just have been.' I wondered if she had been worried about sharing with her boyfriend and his sister. 'Not at first but then she said her man had had hep and I thought if she's sharing with me then she's sharing with him.'

(Hospital detoxification unit)

In this situation the woman had been previously sharing injecting equipment with her boyfriend without perceiving it as particularly risky. However, on finding out that her boyfriend was also sharing injecting equipment with his sister, whose partner had had hepatitis, she began to perceive the possible risks involved and from that point on began to use only her own injecting equipment.

The distinction between theme and horizon may explain how some sharing occurs even though an individual may know the risks involved. This distinction can only offer a *partial* explanation though. There were numerous occasions in our data when drug injectors shared injecting equipment even though they not only knew the risks, but perceived those risks within the particular situation. To explain such occasions it is worthwhile considering further aspects of Schutz's work on the phenomenology of everyday social life.

According to Schutz one of the characteristic features of everyday social life is that for the most part it is a largely taken for granted universe. However, whilst being largely taken for granted, individuals are also constantly engaged in noticing, planning, organizing and acting upon particular aspects of their everyday world. For an aspect of one's everyday world to become thematic it is necessary, Schutz suggests, for it to have become topically relevant. Elements within one's social world may become topically relevant either because an individual freely chooses to focus upon a particular aspect, or as a result of an external influence. For example, sharing injecting equipment might become topically relevant because that person begins to think about the risks of HIV infection (intrinsic relevance) or as a result of having been recently counselled as to the dangers of sharing (imposed relevance). Schutz uses the term motivational relevance to point to the set of interests which guide the individual in influencing those aspects of his or her world which become topically relevant. For example, if an individual finds out that his or her sexual partner has been diagnosed HIV positive this may lead the individual to be much more aware of HIV than in the past and may mean that he or she assesses the risks of sharing differently. In this sense the risks of HIV infection could be said to have become motivationally relevant for the individual.

According to Schutz (1970), how one actually behaves in relation to whichever aspect of one's everyday world is topically relevant will depend upon one's interpretational relevance. Within everyday life, Schutz suggests, interpretation takes place by comparing one's current situation with any typically similar situation in one's past. One recognizes that the situation is of such and such nature by comparing it with similar past experiences. Deciding how to act in a situation is closely tied to interpretation. By reviewing one's past experience the individual identifies not only similar situations, but also stock recipes for how those similar situations were dealt with. The sort of recipes which one has within one's stock of knowledge are influenced by one's motivational relevance. For example, if AIDS and HIV have become prominent parts of one's motivational relevance it is likely that specific recipes will have been devised for coping with situations where there is a risk of HIV transmission. A good illustration of this can be seen in the way in which HIV positive drug injectors often seemed to have developed standard ways of responding to requests to share their injecting equipment:

> I asked Helen (HIV positive injector) about lending equipment. 'There's no way I'd do it. I wouldn't wish this on ma worst enemy. I've been asked for ma works but I just say no and they'll say "how can you no help me, I'm pure strung out" and I'll say "look I've no' got the virus but I don't know about you so I'm no' sharin ma tools".'
>
> (HIV counselling clinic)

Where AIDS and HIV are not so motivationally relevant it is less likely that the individual will have developed a standard recipe to respond to such requests. We have illustrated Schutz's schema in Figure 1. The important question we need to ask is whether this schema can help us in explaining sharing in terms of the factors identified in the previous section.

First, as we noted earlier not all of the drug injectors we contacted were concerned with the risks of HIV. A few, for example, believed themselves to be immune from infection whilst others seemed fatalistic, believing that there was nothing one could do to avoid becoming infected if that was one's destiny. In this sense we would say that AIDS and HIV were not

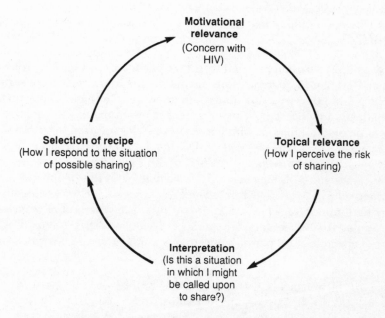

Figure 1   Schutz's schema of systems of relevance

Source: Schutz, A. (1970) *Reflections on the Problem of Relevance.* New York and London, Yale
University Press.

motivationally relevant for that person and he or she might share on a
regular basis with very little attempt at risk reduction.

Second, although at an analytic level one might be able to identify a
single motivational relevance, for example, a concern with AIDS and HIV,
in practice it is likely that there will be a number of different and in some
situations competing motivational relevances. For example, AIDS and HIV
may have become motivationally relevant to an individual, and in the light
of this he or she might be able to cope adequately with requests to share
injecting equipment from a relative stranger. Where such a request comes
from a close friend or sexual partner, however, responding in this way may
be more difficult. Within this latter situation the associated rights and
obligations of friendship may provide a different and more influential set of
motivational relevances bearing on the decision to share:

Anya asked if she could have an extra needle and syringe for her
friend. 'she borrowed ma works this afternoon, she's clean y'know,
she got the test done and it came back clear but still. I took ma hit,
then she took hers, that was the last hit. See, I can't really bleach them
in front of her can I? It'll offend her, y'know, she's ma pal so it's

hard, she'll look at me funny if I get the bleach out, so I just put them
in the drawer, left them like that.'

(Red-light district)

Equally, an individual might begin to experience the effects of drug withdrawal and a desire to overcome this discomfort might override a concern
with AIDS and HIV. In a situation where there is a shortage of injecting
equipment an individual might share rather than postpone his or her drug
use and prolong the effects of withdrawal. Within this situation the motivational relevance of a concern with AIDS and HIV may have been supplanted by a concern to reduce the effects of drug withdrawal.

Third, although AIDS may be motivationally relevant for the individual,
and sharing may have become topically relevant; nevertheless, the individual may find him or herself in a situation in which new topical relevances
may be imposed. One situation where this can be seen is where other drug
injectors demand to use a person's injecting equipment, perhaps with associated threats:

Earlier on in our chat Clive had said that he had recently been in
prison. I asked if he had hit up then and he stated emphatically that
there's more drugs in prison than out and proceeded to demonstrate
how you could conceal drugs on your person following a visit. I asked
him if he had shared works and he said no, that he had had his own set
hidden, explaining that had other prisoners known of his works they
would have asked him for a loan 'and you cannae turn them down'.

(Hospital detoxification unit)

Within such a situation the topically relevant concern to avoid sharing may
be supplanted by the new topically relevant concern with avoiding physical
assault. The individual may be obliged to pass on injecting equipment even
whilst preferring not to.

Fourth, AIDS may have become motivationally relevant, sharing may
have become topically relevant and yet the individual might fail to interpret
correctly a situation as one in which sharing might occur. Confusion arising
as to the ownership of equipment may be seen as an instance of the
individual's failure to interpret correctly the situation as one in which
sharing was likely to occur.

Fifth, AIDS and HIV may have become motivationally relevant, sharing
might also have become topically relevant. The situation may have been
correctly interpreted as one in which he or she might be asked to share, yet
the recipe selected for coping with this request might be inadequate:

We had a discussion about people refusing to take things from drug
injectors because of a fear of AIDS – like canned drinks. Harry
quipped 'I hate those cunts who want to use your works and you say

you can't, I've got the virus and they say "Well so do I so it doesnae matter".'

(Residential detoxification unit)

Although in the past the individual might have been able to turn down requests to share by claiming to have the virus (truthfully or not), such a recipe is undermined if the person requesting the equipment claims that he or she is also HIV positive. To be able to successfully turn down such a request requires developing a strategy that does not rely for its effectiveness on an assumption that the person requesting the injecting equipment is HIV negative.

The attractiveness of Schutz's schema for each of these situations lies in its ability to explain sharing not in terms of the deviant motivations and intentions of drug injectors, but in terms of drug injectors' real life situations. We noted earlier that one of the most striking features of sharing when seen within the context of drug injectors' lives was precisely how normal that sharing appeared. Schutz's schema preserves that quality by allowing one to explain sharing through reference to that context.

Summary and policy implications

We will summarize this chapter and outline some of the policy implications of our work on sharing.

It is clear that irrespective of the media coverage stressing the risks of sharing, both lending and borrowing of injecting equipment are continuing. By far the greatest proportion of the drug injectors contacted reported being prepared to pass on their equipment if asked to do so. Most of the sharing we identified involved sexual partners, close friends and family members. Situations of group sharing were less frequently reported. There is little doubt that availability of sterile injecting equipment was an important factor influencing the decision to use another's needle and syringe. However, there are other influences at work, most notably accidental sharing, the individual's perceived need to inject, his or her assessment of the likely risks involved, the nature of the relationship involved, and broader social norms within the drug culture. It is the combination of these factors within the context of the drug injector's lifestyle that produce sharing.

Previous attempts to explain sharing have been couched in terms of the deviant motivations of drug injectors or gaps in their knowledge of the risks involved. We feel a better explanation can be found in an examination of the social situations confronted by drug injectors. In this respect, Alfred Schutz's work on the phenomenology of everyday life provides a theoretical schema for explaining how the various identified factors may be combined to produce sharing by some drug injectors and not others, and in some situations and not others.

In terms of the policy implications of our work, we would stress three points. First, there is a clear need in health education campaigns to focus attention on the dangers of borrowing *and* lending. A two-pronged approach aimed at both activities is likely to be more successful than one which concentrates only on borrowing, as has been the case in the past.

Second, it seems likely that some sharing will persist irrespective of whatever health education campaigns are implemented. This seems particularly likely where sharing is a feature of drug injectors' relationships or the broader culture within the local area. In the light of this, drug injectors should be encouraged to sterilize their needles and syringes, and if necessary, provided with the means for doing so (household bleach). Such an approach has been successfully implemented in a number of North American cities (Broadhead and Fox 1990). There is a particular case to implement this measure within such institutional settings as prisons and residential drug detoxification units where it is inconceivable that sterile injecting equipment would ever be made available. To provide bleach in this way will undoubtedly be seen by some as condoning drug use within those settings. However, there is a need to consider the possibility that without such a measure both settings may be more effective at spreading HIV infection than they are at treating drug addiction or responding to criminality. To encourage the practice of sterilization within a context where sharing occurs between friends, family and sexual partners is also likely to be difficult. However, this measure would go some way to reducing the risks involved where sharing is going to take place.

Third, whilst government campaigns stressing the message 'Don't Share' may be successful in increasing public awareness of the dangers of sharing, drug injectors will undoubtedly continue to share unless they are provided with the means for changing their behaviour. In addition to providing easier access to sterile injecting equipment, it would be valuable to provide drug injectors with the interactional means (recipes) through social skills training, to enable them to recognize and avoid situations in which sharing is likely to occur, and to be able to turn down requests to share without feeling that they are simultaneously compromising their personal or social relationships with others.

In the next chapter we will shift our focus and look in detail at the sexual behaviour of drug injectors and the risks this might pose for the future spread of HIV infection.

Chapter 4

Drug injectors and the heterosexual spread of HIV infection

Introduction

In this chapter we look at the related issues of heterosexual transmission of HIV infection and the practice of safer sex, particularly with regard to the use of condoms. First, we look at sexual activity and levels of condom use among those drug injectors with whom we were in contact. This provides an important frame of reference for discussing the range of reasons which might impinge upon sexual practice and condom use. We identify four main areas which may be influential in relation to condom use and safer sex. These are: perceptions of risk of heterosexually acquiring the virus; the processes leading up to the sexual encounter; notions of gender appropriate behaviour; and long-term relationships. In the interests of providing a broader perspective on sexual behaviour and attitudes, drug injectors and non-drug injectors alike form the focus of discussion. This was motivated by finding that issues relating to sex and safer sex were no more easily spoken about, dealt with or resolved by drug injectors than they were by those young people we contacted who were not injecting drugs.

Sexual activity and levels of condom use

Safer sex generally refers to the use of condoms as a means of protecting against the exchange of body fluids which might be infected with HIV. Clearly, the best protection against HIV would be to avoid sex altogether and failing that to avoid penetrative sex. However, to expect this degree of behaviour change is unrealistic, not least because sexual expression is generally regarded as a fundamental feature of human relationships. The majority of men and women drug injectors in this study were no different in this respect; they too in the main reported being sexually active. It is worth noting that the use of drugs like Temgesic (buprenorphine), the main drug of use in Glasgow (Sakol *et al.* 1989), does not appear to repress libido in the same way as heroin is reputed to do. Indeed those few who reported being sexually inactive tended to explain it in terms of a specific addiction to heroin:

'. . . with the junk, sex is the last thing on your mind.'

(Needle exchange)

'. . . tae tell ye the truth, smack takes over fae sex, it's smack ye love.'

(Needle exchange)

'. . . I don't bother wi' sex, I just get ma hit, go to ma house, get ma sleep, wake up and have ma hit, like that.'

(Needle exchange)

Despite health educationalists' efforts to encourage heterosexuals to avoid penetrative sex, it is clear that other sexual practices, such as for example, mutual masturbation, if they happen at all, are not generally regarded as substitutes for penetration. Indeed, they appear to be seen as a part of the process leading up to penetration, the act which for many people defines sexual intercourse (Kent *et al.* 1990).

Contrary to popular stereotypes of drug injectors as deviant in every respect, including the realm of sexual behaviour, the great majority of the individuals we interviewed were apparently sexually conservative. A similar finding has recently been reported in a study of drug injectors and their sexual partners in New York (Kane 1991). Most of the drug injectors were in long-term sexual relationships with one partner, only a minority self-identified as homosexual or lesbian. Again, only a very small number of people reported having had many casual sexual contacts, such as, for example, the following reported behaviour:

'Aye, well I'm very promiscuous and I have slept with women who are HIV positive without a condom'. He later estimated having slept with about 9 women in the last two weeks.

(Needle exchange)

Tom said he'd slept with a good few women, some drug injectors, some he felt had the virus. 'That's what I'm afraid of, in case I catch it through the thingummy . . . the willie, the penis. . . . I just cannae resist they women'.

(Residential detoxification unit)

Even a few such individuals, however, have the potential to generate epidemic spread. The finding of a small number of people, mainly men, who report large numbers of casual sexual contacts is in keeping with recent research on drug injectors attending needle exchanges in England and Scotland (Donoghoe *et al*. 1989).

Both our own study and that of Donoghoe and his colleagues (1989) found that the overwhelming majority of male injectors had sexual partners who did not themselves inject drugs. Undoubtedly, part of the reason for this is simple arithmetic; there are many more men using drugs than there are women using them. A recently reported figure shows a ratio of 2.5 male to 1 female drug user in Glasgow (Frischer *et al*. 1991). This finding can also be explained by an oft stated preference amongst the male injectors for women not using drugs:

Tam said he wouldn't go out with a girl who was using drugs. 'I don't know why but I don't like to see a girl using, you know puttin' a needle in her arm, I don't think a girl should do that. I suppose a man shouldnae either, but somehow its worse in a girl, aye, a girl wi' a wean'.

(Needle exchange)

He expressed distaste for having a woman who was also using drugs 'It wouldnae be long before she'd be workin' down that town (prostituting) and I couldnae handle that, it's degrading'.

(Residential detoxification unit)

The commonest explanation for this preference for women not injecting drugs was moral in character and centred on what was seen as the inappropriateness of a woman injecting. This has also been reported in other studies of women injectors (Rosenbaum 1981; Cohen *et al*. 1989).

It is pragmatic to use condoms as a means of protecting against the exchange of body fluids which may be HIV infected. Condoms do provide a practical and relatively effective means of guarding against HIV infection. There are, however, a number of objections to their use which clearly illustrate the dangers of regarding use of condoms as unproblematical. The main objections to condoms are well known; people report them to be clumsy, messy and unreliable as a contraceptive measure, as well as being embarrassing and difficult to negotiate. The problems associated with condom use pre-date the advent of HIV infection (Wellings 1988).

A particular objection often raised by men is that condoms are desensitizing, a feeling articulated by this male drug injector who claimed to have large numbers of sexual contacts:

'D'ye want me to carry condoms wi' me? You'd be as well havin' sex wi' a tea cosy on.' I quizzed James further over his saying that he worried about his sexual contacts with women he felt were 'dodgy', what did that worry mean in practice? 'After it (sexual intercourse) you're like that for a wee while: "Jeez what have I fuckin' done ?".'

He ended by saying that he felt that sex with a condom was a waste of time, 'better off reading a book'.

(Residential detoxification unit)

A factor influencing use of condoms which may be more specific to drug injectors than others relates to the effects of some of the drugs used. The injected use of temazepam is a case in point as this is often associated with lack of control and awareness (Klee *et al.* 1990). Some of the people interviewed said that they had felt too 'stoned' to think about anything very much:

I asked Kate if she'd used condoms with her last sexual partner 'No, we were both too full o' it'.

(Hospital detoxification unit)

It is evident that condoms remain generally unpopular, as this non-drug using man commented:

'. . . there's 15 reasons why people won't use them, at least 15 reasons, one reason and that just discourages them altogether, from things like buying them to wearing them, anything, and I don't think there is enough done by the government to promote it, maybe it's not a good thing to promote but it is good, it's not sort of the done thing.'

(Community centre)

The unpopularity of condoms, whether for purposes of preventing conception or preventing possible transmission of the virus is illustrated in Table 3.

Table 3   Condom use

	Needle exchange ($n = 40$)	Chemist ($n = 83$)	Total ($n = 123$)
Using condom	15 (37.5%)	18 (21.7%)	33 (26.8%)
Not using condom	25 (62.5%)	65 (78.3%)	90 (73.2%)

Out of a total of 123 drug injecting men and women interviewed in both the pharmacy and the needle exchange, only 26 per cent reported the use of condoms. Amongst the small number of people who reported consistently using condoms, the rationale for their use was most often framed in terms of a concern to avoid HIV infection rather than for purposes of avoiding conception:

'I'm careful, I always carry a condom. I have one on me the now 'cos you never know.' He said he didn't have a girlfriend at the moment but of the last three partners, two had been users.

(Needle exchange)

'Ma boyfriend who hits up and me always use condoms 'cos I wouldnae know if he had slept around or used someone else's tools.'

(Pharmacy)

Others reported using condoms inconsistently, depending on whether or not they were available at the time:

I asked him if he thought that he might be at risk of HIV through his sexual contacts: 'I use condoms, well not every time right enough. If I don't have any on me then I'll do without them. I'm no' bothered about usin' one though. I don't like them but I use them.'

(Needle exchange)

Despite repeated campaigns stressing the importance of condom use it is clear that their use remains problematic. To understand the reasons behind the low take-up rate of condoms it is important to place the issue of their use within the context of the social relationships of which they are a part. Precisely because the use of condoms is a social act and has social meaning it should be credited as being more than a simple mechanical procedure (Weinstein and Goebel 1979).

The following sections will look in more detail at the range of factors which influenced the use of condoms.

Perceptions of risk

A first step towards preventing risk behaviour is to inform people of the risks involved in the behaviours one wishes to change. Since 1987 successive health education campaigns have stressed the risks of heterosexual transmission of the virus. However, research into the effects of these campaigns, with the notable exception of the 1988 National Survey of Adolescent Males in North America, suggests very little behaviour change, (Sonenstein et al. 1989). In this country at least many heterosexuals appear unconvinced that they might themselves be at risk of HIV infection via heterosexual sex (Nutbeam 1989; Macdonald and Smith 1990). This appears to hold true as much among the drug injectors as in the population generally (Donoghoe et al. 1989; Klee 1990). The following field extracts are illustrative of the range of responses given:

'Aye I do worry (about sexual transmission of the virus), but I've heard that it's difficult for a guy to get it fae a lassie.'

(Needle exchange)

In reply to my question as to whether or not he used condoms, John answered 'I've nae need of them, I've been tested and I'm negative.' The charge nurse then asked about his partner; 'I've just the one bird and she's nae junkie.'

(Needle exchange)

Neil asked if he would use condoms, he shook his head; 'nah, I'd know if the bird was sleepin' around.'

(Pharmacy)

Furthermore, it was often demonstrated that the risks of sexual transmission were not considered anything like as serious as the risks of infection through sharing used needles and syringes:

Each time I bring up the subject of condoms and unprotected sex I draw a blank. They seem to see the issue as totally unrelated to them.

(Residential detoxification unit)

It became apparent during the course of this study that most people found it difficult to sustain an image of themselves as potentially infected and, therefore, a risk to other people. More commonly they saw themselves as at risk from others. As a result sexual transmission of the virus tended to be discussed in terms of the likelihood that they would become infected rather than in terms of them passing on HIV infection to their sexual partners. This may partly be as a result of health education campaigns which have tended to emphasize the risk of becoming infected rather than the risk of passing infection on to others. However, this is somewhat ironic in the case of the large numbers of men whose sexual partners were most often women who were not injecting drugs:

'No you can't really get it that way can you? I mean maybe if I had a girlfriend who was usin' I might be worried but apart from that, I'm no' worried.'

(Needle exchange)

Some men had partners who did not know of their injecting drug use. This was also found to be the case in a study in New York (Kane 1991). Clearly, this is a piece of information which is relevant in assessing one's personal risk of HIV infection and might have been instrumental in deciding on the value of using condoms. Being in possession of the facts is yet more relevant where a potential partner has the virus:

Tina described the first time she and Tim (HIV positive) got together. '. . . I don't drink really but that night I was steamin'. Well that night we slept wi' each other and we didnae use a condom or anything. Then next day I heard he had a hospital appointment and then I twigged. He wasnae steamin' he knew what he was doin' and he had the virus and he didnae even tell me. That really hurt me.'

(Streetwork field-note)

The fact of the other person's HIV seropositivity might, in the event, not be the deciding factor in terms of whether barrier protection is used or even if sexual intercourse takes place. Nonetheless, it is information that is of significance to the other person. However, our contacts with people who had HIV or other infections which could be sexually transmitted illustrated the very real difficulties which might be experienced in revealing the fact of being infected:

> Tracey talked about her ex-boyfriend saying she still likes him but doesn't know what to do if she goes out with him again because of her hepatitis. 'I mean how can I ask him to use a condom, say I don't want to get pregnant? I don't want him to know about this hep but I don't want him to get it.'
>
> (Residential detoxification unit)

Even suggesting the use of a condom could be interpreted as indicating that one was HIV positive oneself or that one suspected that one's partner might be. Clearly, this can create problems:

> 'One lassie she said to me "you'll need to wear one o' them" but after I think she felt bad, like her conscience was guilty that she thought she might get something off me, but I said "no, you're right, you're right to be careful".'
>
> (Needle exchange)

A central tenet of health education campaigns has been to communicate the message that a person with asymptomatic HIV infection looks exactly the same as anybody else. It was evident though that many of the people we spoke to felt they could tell if someone was HIV infected from their physical appearance:

> I asked him if he knew anyone who was HIV positive and he said he didn't. At this point he started asking me about the symptoms of HIV/ AIDS and began pinching his face, asking me if I thought he looked thin and unhealthy.
>
> (Hospital detoxification unit)

> 'You can tell if someone's got the virus, know how you can tell? Their faces and bodies are dead, dead thin, pure wasted, but around here (she slapped her thigh) they're like that (big), that's the only place they don't lose it. That's how you can tell if someone's got the virus.'
>
> (Needle exchange)

The tendency of people to associate HIV infection with an unhealthy or unkempt appearance has also been reported in another Glasgow based study (Kitzinger 1990). The problem is that if physical attraction is at least partly defined in terms of appearances (of which presumably 'cleanliness' is a component part), then the issue of whether or not the potential sexual partner is HIV infected is already likely to have been discounted. Following through the logic of this assessment there is then no obvious need to use a condom. This much seems the case from the schoolboys' evaluations of when to use a condom:

> I asked if they would insist on condom use, the girls were unanimous, the boys less certain all shaking their heads. So I asked: 'You wouldn't wear one then?' 'Nah, no' if I'd been goin' with her a while', 'depends if she was boggin'.

> (School)

It may be that part of the decision as to whether or not safer sex is even worth considering is still premised on evaluating the appearance of the person in whom one is sexually interested.

Broadly, the same external criteria employed by drug injectors to decide if someone was HIV positive were also employed by the non-drug users to identify people injecting drugs. Although some did say that you might not always be able to tell if someone was injecting drugs, in general most of the non-injectors were confident that you could tell either by the thinness of injectors, or by looking at their eyes; 'their eyes go all funny', or the pallor of their skin; 'they go all white after a while'. Apart from this there was agreement that drug injectors could be identified by their shabby dress and unkempt appearance.

The schoolchildren we spoke to appeared to rely on external cues to identify drug injectors. One reason for this was because direct enquiry about another's involvement in drugs was seen as socially unacceptable:

> We asked if they'd ask if she/he was using drugs. 'No, you wouldnae ask them'. This was the general feeling – besides they all felt sure you could tell without asking. It was felt to be insulting to ask someone if they were, even if you were going to have sex with them and anyway if you were 'you'd know them by then enough to know if they were a junkie.'

> (School)

The overall impression we received from our contacts with people who did not inject drugs was a certainty that they would be able to detect if someone was injecting drugs before becoming either sexually or emotionally involved with them. It is, however, noteworthy that in this study many of the women who began injecting in the context of a sexual relationship first became involved with men who were injecting unbeknownst to them. Similarly, in a New York study (Kane 1991) most sex partners did not know that their partner was injecting drugs until well after the relationship was established.

Negotiating the sexual encounter and safer sex

Efforts to encourage widespread use of condoms are hampered in our society by the fact that issues of sex and sexuality have all the trappings of a taboo subject (Mittag 1991). Only rarely is sex a subject of conversation in any meaningful sense, most often issues relating to it are swathed in ambiguity, awkwardness and uncertainty. This perhaps explains the paucity of our vocabulary for expressing these concerns in ways which are not themselves charged with sexual meaning or innuendo, or so oblique as to lose all meaning. One consequence of this observed cultural reticence to raise the subject of sex and discuss it frankly is that we know very little about sexual behaviour. From the point of view of health educationalists this creates the obvious difficulty of targetting appropriate strategies aimed at changing behaviours.

The difficulties associated with raising the subject of sex as a matter for open discussion were very apparent during our fieldwork. Whilst the risks of HIV transmission through shared needles were frequently discussed in detail and at length, the risks of sexual transmission were relatively rarely discussed and never in great detail. Men and women alike often mentioned being embarrassed to talk in depth about sexual matters and finding it difficult to discuss the subject without awkwardness. This was well illustrated during the group discussions in the schools:

> 'So', I probed, 'what other way can you get the virus apart from sharing needles/blood?' A coy answer from one girl 'through sleeping with someone', a ripple of embarrassed laughter spread through the group. 'How can you protect yourself?' I asked. Again a certain coyness and one boy in saying 'condoms' provoked much laughter.
>
> (School)

Although to differing degrees, depending on whether or not we spoke to people in groups or alone, this same awkwardness and embarrassment was apparent in all of the settings in which we contacted people. It is also worth noting that there were times when we unconsciously colluded in a number of ways with this reticence to discuss issues of sex. In retrospect it often seems that an unwarranted sensitivity on our part was brought to bear on the research situation, such that the subject of sex was not probed further if the person concerned seemed uncomfortable with the subject. Additionally, the subject of sex was often ruled out of bounds by the nature of the situation. Discussions of heterosexual risks of HIV infection are, for example, conspicuously absent from our contacts with drug injectors in public settings. It would seem that the researchers and their subjects were adhering to a mutual understanding of the appropriateness of certain settings for certain subjects. The issue of when, where and how to address potentially sensitive subjects has surfaced in other research work such as that reported by Stimson and his colleagues (1988).

The view that sexual behaviour is a private, personal concern appears culturally embedded in our society. The fact that issues concerning sex do not appear to be raised often for discussion even between sexual partners further suggests the extraordinary status of sex in our society (Mittag 1991). Clearly, sex is treated as something to be negotiated with care and due caution. Recognizing the delicacy and complexity of the processes involved in the negotiation of the sexual encounter is an essential part of understanding the many influences which cut across the seemingly straightforward injunction of health educationalists to ensure against sexual spread of the virus by encouraging condom use.

The term 'negotiation of safer sex' has been much used in recent years to help foster an awareness of the preventable risks of HIV infection in sexual encounters. However, for many the term bears little relationship to the realities of sexual experience in which the negotiation of any kind of sex, let alone the use of condoms, might be considered a hazardous, uncertain and potentially fraught business (Barnard and McKeganey 1990; Brooks–Gunn and Furstenberg 1990).

Although there has been little systematic work in this area, it appears that ambiguity is an important feature of the process leading up to sexual relations between heterosexuals (Kent *et al.* 1990). Given the importance that is generally attached to sex in human relationships this is perhaps not surprising. It does, however, present certain difficulties in so far as the introduction of safer sex practices are concerned. The problem is that negotiating safer sex requires a degree of explicitness which may actually be in opposition to the whole tenor of the proceedings.

The lead up to sexual relations appears to be one of an incremental process signposted by mutually understood if non-verbal signals which represent a gradual move towards a situation where agreement to sexual relations is taken to be consensual. By avoiding making explicit statements of sexual intent both parties may be able to avoid potential embarrassment or discomfort should the advances of either be rejected. Physical signs such as switching off the light or locking the door are often used to represent the wish to take things one step further. If the other person consents to this turn of events, this may then be read as agreement to have sex. The overriding impression is one of a progressive move towards a situation in which sex 'becomes' the agenda, even if this is never explicitly acknowledged by those involved. It is almost as if a necessary fiction is created such that the actual consummation of the sex act is frequently represented as a spontaneous, unported event, although it can be seen analytically as the result of a protracted, careful and subtle process of negotiation.

The point at which it is 'decided' between two people (whether overtly or not) that they will have sexual relations appears to mark the end of the negotiating process. Consummation may follow on very quickly from this point. In terms of the structure of the process it would appear that it is only really in the compressed space between agreement and consummation that the issue of safer sex could be introduced. This itself creates a number of problems as the ambiguity inherent in the process of preparing the way for sexual relations, by its nature, does not allow for explicit recognition of intent; discussing safer sex at this point would be to place the cart before the horse. However, to raise the issue once it is agreed that sex is on the agenda may not be particularly easy either, this much is apparent from the following field-notes:

> Bill reminded Tim of a time when Sam was trying to get a condom out of the machine. The laugh seemed to be that he'd paid £1 for one condom. I asked if it was worth it and Sam said he hadn't used it. Bill interpreted it to mean that it was hard to use a condom when you were in the middle of it. Sam agreed saying there was no way he was going to stop to put a rubber on, 'cause if you do you'll lose it'.
>
> (Street field-note)

> He thinks he may have the virus (although earlier on he'd said he didn't think so) because he's slept around. I asked if he knew how many partners he'd had, 'oh millions and I never used a condom. When you're in the bedroom you're not thinking about a condom, only one thing on your mind then.'
>
> (Hospital detoxification unit)

In both cases it would seem as if there is no room for further negotiation, sex had become the main agenda.

Women bargaining from a position of weakness?

Traditional gender-related expectations of behaviour places the onus upon men to take the lead in initiating sexual relationships with women (Jackson 1982; Richardson 1990). In this society at least, it would appear that male dominance is an expected feature of the heterosexual relationship. This can effectively place limits on the woman's potential to negotiate with her partner over the issue of safer sex (Holland *et al.* 1990b). Given societal expectations of female passivity and the additional expectation that a woman should not profess to know too much about sex (James *et al.* 1979), a woman might feel unable to raise the issue of condom use without inviting negative comment (Pollack 1985). This seems apparent in the following field extract; even though the woman was asking the researcher for condoms, her whole manner suggested real difficulty in insisting on their use:

> I asked Jenna if she worried about getting HIV through sexual relations. 'I do, that's how I'm gettin' condoms fae you' (she whispered

this to me, her boyfriend was nearby and she didn't want him to hear).
'He doesnae want tae use them but I think he should because like I
says to him, "I don't know who youse are with and if youse are sharin'
their tools and sleepin' wi' girls, I've got tae protect ma health, think
of myself".'

(Needle exchange)

In the context of a cultural expectation of female naivety about sex it
might be considered inappropriate for her to be in possession of a condom
(Scott 1987). Certainly, the schoolchildren in our study were sensitive to
these issues. Despite the girls' greater professed willingness to use condoms
as barrier protection they were sensitive to the moral comment which
might possibly attach to them carrying condoms:

The girls all said they'd be embarrassed to carry a condom and said
their friends would think they were a slag if they found out they were
carrying one.

(School)

Not surprisingly, this same reticence to carry condoms was also noted
among female drug injectors:

Neil asked if she'd consider using a condom with her next partner.
She seemed unsure. He gave her a hypothetical situation – at a party
and wanting to have sex with a man she'd met there: 'In that situation,
aye.' She then went on to say that they were horrible things and she
wouldn't carry them on her.

(Hospital detoxification unit)

It was interesting to note that many of the schoolboys saw it as the
responsibility of women to carry condoms. This attitude may relate to the
general expectation that women should take charge of contraception to
avoid falling pregnant. The problem, however, is that women are also
supposed to be the guardians of their own morality defending their hon-
our against the onslaught of male desire (Horowitz 1981). A woman who
is seen to be sexually available risks losing her reputation and being
labelled a 'slag' or a 'whore' (James 1986). Clearly, the inclination of
women to carry condoms must be compromised where they stand to be
so poorly judged for doing so. Currently the thrust of a good deal of
health education has been to encourage men and women alike to carry
condoms routinely in order to meet situations where sex becomes the
agenda. However, it is apparent from this study and others (Abrams *et al.*
1990; Barnard and McKeganey 1990) that women, although more prepared to *use* a condom were not prepared to *carry* them for fear of adverse
social comment for doing so.

Condom use in long-term relationships

It could be argued that much of what has been said so far is largely relevant to either new or casual sexual encounters. In making this case, however, it is assumed that sex the second or third time with the same person will be a less uncertain and delicate affair. Recent findings from a study of young people's sexual behaviour though suggest that issues relating to sex are not always raised or resolved between couples in longer term relationships (D. Wight, personal communication).

There are particular problems associated with encouraging the introduction of safer sex practices into long-term relationships. Perhaps the first point to note is that condom use, if it occurs at all, is most often at the start of a relationship. Once it is established that the relationship will continue it is often the case that the woman begins to use the pill for contraception (Holland *et al.* 1990a). Condoms appear to be seen as a temporary measure associated more with the one-off sexual encounters than stable long-term relationships. Liebow reports a similar finding in a pre-AIDS (and pre-pill) study of street corner boys (1967). They were also reluctant to use condoms in their long-term relationships even though they were quite prepared to use them for one-off sexual encounters. This woman commented in the context of the Glasgow study:

> 'There's got to be a time when you get together if you are close and condoms will go out the windae, you know what I mean, that you are not prepared for what is gonnae happen.'
>
> (Residential detoxification unit)

Indeed, there is a degree to which a woman's use of the pill can be taken as signifying commitment or seriousness to the relationship (Kent *et al.* 1990). This seems borne out by the following field extract:

> I asked Joanne if she used condoms with her boyfriend. 'No, I'm gettin' married in a month. I used condoms at first but no' now.' (They have been going out for a year.)
>
> (Pharmacy)

It would appear from this woman's response that condom use was inappropriate at this stage of the relationship. It may well be that the point at which a relationship appears to take on a more stable character is also the point at which condoms are rejected in favour of a less obtrusive form of contraception.

The introduction of condom use into an already established relationship may be still more problematic, particularly if other means of contraception are being used:

> James has a regular girlfriend. She doesn't use drugs but she knows he

does. I asked him if he worried about sexual transmission. He looked surprised at this and said no. I asked if she wanted him to use condoms 'no, she doesnae need to, she's on the pill'.

(Pharmacy)

In this situation it may be very difficult for the partner not to suspect the motives of the other for suggesting the use of barrier protection. The social ramifications of suggesting condom use may be considerable, introducing an element of distrust and uncertainty into the relationship.

Research looking at communication between partners indicates that certain topics are held to be taboo in close relationships. In essence these topics can be seen as those which are potentially threatening to the status of the relationship. Broadly, these subjects relate to sexual history, current sexual activity outside of the relationship and discussing the current state of the relationship (Baxter and Wilmot 1985). Broaching the subject of condom use and, more generally, safer sex may raise concerns which have remained submerged precisely because they are sensitive and, potentially, may de-stabilize the relationship (Perlmutter Bowen and Michel-Johnson 1989; Kane 1991). It is interesting to note in the following field extract the difficulties this man clearly envisages were he to suggest use of condoms in his long-term relationship, even though he recognizes the risks of sexual transmission of the virus:

'If I have sex wi' a girl I don't know I use condoms. Ma girlfriend doesnae use, no, I don't use condoms wi' her. That would be difficult.'

(Needle exchange)

A major obstacle to the use of condoms in the context of long-trm relationships may closely relate to socially constructed notions of intimacy; condom use appears to run counter to ideas of physical and emotional closeness. Condoms create a barrier between a couple which may be seen to be as much symbolic as physical. Generally, relationships are assumed to be about increasing closeness in both emotional and physical terms, and to introduce condom use into this scenario may be difficult because it seems to create distance rather than reduce it (Gillman and Feldman 1991).

Women, perhaps more than men, subscribed to what might be described as the ideology of romantic love such that they often represented themselves as having thrown in their lot with their partner and were ready to face life's trials together:

I asked Jane if she worried at all about AIDS. She was emphatic that she didn't. She injects with the same needle as her boyfriend. 'It doesnae matter, he'll no' share outside and nor will I.' I asked if she and her boyfriend used a condom; 'no, never, there's nae point, what he gets I'll get and same wi' me for him.'

(Residential detoxification unit)

and, in the case of a woman whose boyfriend was HIV positive:

> 'The doctor used to sit and say "you'll have to use them (condoms) because there's nae use you getting it" . . . but I'd just say "och I think I'll be alright" or, "if it happens, it happens." The two of us have got to stay together. I know that sounds weird.'
>
> (Residential detoxification unit)

In the particular case of one's partner being HIV positive it seemed that the non-use of condoms could be a statement of commitment on the part of the other:

> I wondered if being in a relationship with Lenny made it difficult for her to use protection 'You do take chances you know. When it started I fell in love wi' him, and I thought this is forever and ever, and so I didn't think about him wi' the virus and all that much.'
>
> (Streetwork field-note)

The whole issue of safer sex and condom use is clearly at odds with a woman actively seeking to get pregnant (Gillman and Feldman 1991). The following field-note is apposite in this regard:

> 'My boyfriend is usin' (drugs) in the prison just now and I know he's sharin'. No he wouldnae let me use condoms cause he wants to have a wean by me.'
>
> (Pharmacy)

Although aware of her boyfriend's risk behaviour and the consequences this might have for her, this woman felt unable to protect herself against sexual transmission because of her boyfriend's injunction that she get pregnant. More broadly, however, women injectors are socially stigmatized for their involvement in drug use. Generally, they are seen to be in breach of their proper social role. For many women injectors having a child and becoming a mother is one way in which they can aspire to traditional expectations of appropriate female behaviour. Becoming pregnant may, in their terms, come to assume greater importance than using a condom to avoid possible HIV transmission (Mitchell 1988).

Summary and policy implications

Despite successive health education campaigns to encourage condom use as a means of preventing HIV transmission, it is apparent that they remain unpopular as much amongst drug injectors as the population generally. In this chapter we looked at the various reported obstacles or objections to their use. We paid particular attention to the social dimensions of condom use in sexual relationships. As with each of the main chapters in this book we will close by considering some of the policy implications of these findings.

A first important point concerns the difficulties encountered in sustaining an image of oneself as potentially infected and, therefore, at risk of passing on HIV infection to another through sexual contact. Given that so many male drug injectors have non-drug injecting partners there is an urgent need for health education initiatives to encourage a greater sense of responsibility towards the well-being of one's sexual partners. Equal emphasis on the risks of passing on the virus and the risks of contracting it might have the effect of promoting greater condom use.

It is evident from our study and numerous others that condom use is problematical for the majority of people and the reasons for this are largely social in nature. Condom use is not a neutral activity, on the contrary, it appears loaded with meanings which are closely tied to social constructions of sexuality and norms of its expression, to ideas of gender appropriate behaviour and to social circumstance. All of these factors in varying degrees affect the likelihood of condoms being used. Encouraging greater use of condoms must take these factors into account. Admittedly, this is a far from easy task if only because sexual behaviour is so complex and private an affair. Our work suggests that the likelihood of condoms being used is linked to the nature of the relationship itself. Whereas condoms might be used in one-off or infrequent sexual encounters they tend not to be a feature of longer term, regular relationships. This suggests that, for these people, other means of preventing potential HIV transmission may need to be encouraged. Where the use of barrier protection is seen as inimical to the interests of the relationship the next best solution is to prevent a situation where HIV infection might be transmitted to either partner in the first place. Health education media campaigns might address this issue by emphasizing a sense of responsibility for the well-being of one's sexual partner. This is not to suggest that fidelity or monogamy, or even truthfulness, are the only means of demonstrating responsibility. It may be that one or either of the couple becomes involved in behaviour that has a risk of HIV; taking adequate precautionary steps either to minimize or eliminate those risks is not only to protect oneself against HIV infection, but also anyone else who might subsequently also be at risk.

Our work indicates that for many people sex is an uncertain and often fraught affair which, because of its near taboo status, is a difficult subject to raise for open discussion. Furthermore, the ambiguity which appears to surround the lead up to sexual encounters does not lend itself to the negotiation of safer sex and condom use. Policy makers, particularly where schools are concerned, might consider means of encouraging an openness in matters of sex and sexuality on the assumption that the negotiation of safer sex requires a certain clarity as to the issues concerned as well as the assertiveness and confidence to raise them. The value of this approach has recently been demonstrated in Holland where it has been shown that talking about sex in a frank, unfrightening way encourages assertiveness and responsibility in sexual relationships (Godlee 1990). The use of role play in schools might be valuable in this respect as would be the challenging of stereotypic expectations of appropriate female and male behaviours.

Notions of what is appropriate behaviour for males and females appear to have an important influence on attitudes towards condom use and the likelihood that they will be used. In a situation where females are poorly judged for being seen to carry condoms it is unsurprising that they avoid doing so. Future health education campaigns should address this issue by emphasizing that it is equally the responsibility of men and women to take all possible steps to prevent HIV transmission.

Chapter 5

Prostitution, drugs and HIV-related risk behaviour

Introduction

Media representations of HIV and AIDS have a tendency to replace sober reporting with hysterical headlines. Nowhere is this more apparent than in the multitude of 'death on the streets' type news reports which present prostitutes as a reservoir of infection threatening others. In this chapter, however, we will look in detail at the link between injecting drug use, prostitution and HIV-related risk behaviour. Although much of what we go on to say relates primarily to female prostitution, we will also present some information on male prostitution.

HIV-related risk behaviour patterns are considered in terms of the use of unsterile needles and syringes, and the provision of unsafe sex to clients and also to private sexual partners. We also look at the nature of the relationship established between prostitute and client as a factor influencing the likelihood that condoms will be used, both in terms of the prostitute's ability to assert control over the situation, and also in terms of the place and significance of condoms within these situations. We will close by outlining what we see as the policy implications of our work in this area.

Before looking at the extent of the overlap between male and female prostitution and injecting drug use in Glasgow it will be helpful to outline the method of data collection used for this part of the study.

Method of data collection

At the outset we had intended to collect information on male and female prostitution as part of the contacts we were establishing with drug injectors on the streets and at the various treatment agencies where we were interviewing. In fact, this proved very difficult. While we experienced ver little difficulty in interviewing drug injectors about such topics as needle and syringe sharing, we often found it extremely difficult to shift the discussion on to the topic of sex in general, and male and female prostitution in particular. In retrospect one might have anticipated this since these topics are far from neutral. As an alternative, we decided to try to establish direct contacts with male and female prostitutes within the various localities where they were working. To this end we carried out fieldwork in the city's red-light district. We also spent an extended period of time visiting those settings (principally certain public toilets and parks) where it was known that male prostitutes were working.

As a result of this part of our work we were able to contact 208 female prostitutes (we estimate this to be around half of the total female street-working prostitutes in Glasgow) and 32 male prostitutes (estimated as around half of the total male prostitute population in the city; this figure also includes four men who did not work from the street and were contacted via other means).

In contacting female and male prostitutes we combined a research and a service provider role (Barnard 1991). As well as carrying out short interviews with each of the female and male prostitutes, all of the women were offered condoms, sterile injecting equipment and an advice leaflet on HIV risk reduction, with details of various helping agencies. Similarly, the male prostitutes were offered a variety of condoms suitable for oral and anal sex, and an advice leaflet on HIV risk reduction. As we will show, there was much less of a need to provide the male prostitutes with sterile injecting equipment.

Injecting drug use and prostitution

While many of the male prostitutes we contacted reported using alcohol, smoking marijuana or swallowing tablets, injecting drug use by comparison seemed relatively rare:

> I asked Tommy if he ever injected 'No, never'. He said he'd tried other things like eggs (temazepam) but that he had never injected. I said that I had heard that some of the boys would inject amphetamines from time to time, just to keep going. 'No, never heard of that'.
>
> (Barkham Street toilets)

Only five of the 32 male prostitutes we contacted reported injecting drugs. This figure is noteworthy since most of the male prostitutes were working at a street level which one might have anticipated would be where most of the prostitutes who injected drugs would be working.

Two of the five drug injecting male prostitutes had begun injecting whilst working as prostitutes. Of the three who were injecting prior to prostituting, two had reputations for mugging clients:

> Roddy spoke to us between punters. He repeated a lot of the information he gave us before: about how he started off by rolling punters but found that he couldn't get any custom, about how he hates renting but must have the money for his habit. He's currently using heroin but there's a shortage of Tems and he's not had any for two weeks. He doesn't like using heroin because it is so adulterated. As it is he believes that the chalk in the Tems is responsible for the problems he's been having with his legs where he injects. He bought £30 of heroin yesterday. He's planning to get himself off heroin by buying loads of eggs (temazepam) and blocking off on them until the worst of the withdrawal pangs are passed.
>
> (Arthur Street toilets)

It is worth noting, however, that the practice of demanding or forcibly removing money from clients is not exclusive to those injecting drugs. At least three other rent boys reported demanding money on occasion and yet another had begun his prostitute career by mugging clients (Bloor *et al.* 1991a).

Some of the male prostitutes expressed negative feelings towards those who were prostituting in order to finance a drug habit, others said they found the practice of injecting drug use in itself abhorrent:

> Junkies working as rent boys were a minority he said. He added that he had watched someone hitting up recently and had found it absolutely repulsive – he described in some detail how the junkie had cleaned the puncture marks with a dirty piece of towel.
>
> (Arthur Street toilets)

The low level of injecting drug use amongst the male prostitutes we contacted is in keeping with research carried out in Edinburgh (Morgan Thomas *et al.* 1989) and London (Robinson 1989). In the United States, however, Waldorf and Murphy (1990) report that over half of the male prostitutes they contacted were injecting drug users. One explanation for so little injecting amongst the male prostitutes in Glasgow might be that the sort of money being made by the male prostitutes we contacted was insufficient to finance a drug habit. It was a common occurrence during our fieldwork, for example, to see a male prostitute hanging around a pick-up point for a number of hours without attracting more than a single client.

The briskness of trade for female streetworking prostitutes afforded a vivid contrast to the situation for streetworking rent boys. Women were seen frequently stepping in and out of cars, and there was no obvious shortage of punters. Since the streetworking males only obtained between

£5 and £15 ($9–27) per client (in London the rates are between £20 and £25), it is difficult to see how they would have been able to support a drug habit from prostituting alone. The apparent irregularity of the income which prostitution generated, along with the physical deterioration associated with injecting drug use (clients place a premium on youthful good looks) may have been further reasons why there was so little injecting amongst the male prostitutes we contacted:

> On arrival Mike was talking to Malcolm. I was surprised since I hadn't seen Mike for a couple of months (in that time he had begun injecting drugs and was also homeless) the change in him was dramatic, Marina and I were both shocked by it. His skin was pallid, drawn and spotty; there were old bruises on his face; his eyes were sunken and heavy lidded; his movements were slow; he stank and his clothes were dirty. The transformation from the cocky wise-cracking Mike of old was total; no more bragging about high-spending punters and the sharp clothes they'd bought him.
>
> (Arthur Street toilets)

The situation in relation to the female streetworking prostitutes we contacted was the diametric opposite of that for the male prostitutes in almost every respect. In Table 4 we have summarized our information on drug injecting amongst the 208 female streetworking prostitutes interviewed:

Table 4 Female streetworking prostitution and injecting drug use

	Number of individuals	Number of contacts
Drug injectors	122	354
	(58.7%)	(66.7%)
Non-injectors	86	177
	(41.3%)	(33.3%)
Total	208	531

Almost 60 per cent of the female streetworking prostitutes contacted were injecting drug users. This figure is considerably higher than has been reported for other cities in Britain (Day 1988; Kinnell 1989; Morgan Thomas *et al.* 1989). What partially explains this is our sole concentration on streetworking women. This contrasts with other studies which have tended to combine together various different styles of prostitute work, for example, streetworking women, and women working saunas and massage parlours. Most studies have shown higher proportions of injecting among those women working on the streets. Certainly, some of the women we were in contact with provided us with accounts of sauna and massage parlour owners checking the women for any evidence of drug injecting:

> Judy started to get worried about the track marks on her arms. She'd tried to inject last week and had a sizeable bruise on her arm. She also had a series of scabs which followed her vein on her arm. She said that the woman at the sauna had told her she wouldn't accept her if she was a junkie. She'd noticed the bruise on Judy's arm but Judy had told her it was from the hospital and that she had a kidney problem. She tried to cover the track marks by using a plaster but both Jimmy (boyfriend) and I felt that drew attention to it, so we covered her arm with foundation cream instead. Jimmy said that she should say that she had been battered by him. Judy though said 'what kind of a man will they think you are if I say that?'
>
> (Streetwork field-note)

Although our finding that nearly 60 per cent of streetworking women were injecting drug users is indicative of the potential risks of HIV transmission, it is likely to be an underestimate of the actual situation. For instance, although only one of the non-drug injecting women reported prostituting to finance her sexual partner's drug injecting habit, it represents an HIV transmission risk similar to those of women who were prostituting to finance their own drug use. In addition, it seems highly likely that some of the women we classified as non-injectors were, in fact, injecting, but had concealed this from us. Furthermore, those women who were prostituting in order to finance their own drug use appeared to be working more frequently and for longer hours than their non-drug injecting counterparts. On more than a third of the nights we carried out fieldwork in the red light area, for example, drug injecting women amounted to more than 75 per cent of the total women seen working.

Women who become involved in prostitution quickly find themselves earning sums of money far in excess of that which they could legitimately earn. The field-note below is an apt illustration of this earning power:

> Tracy exampled the kind of money she was making. 'I got £100 the other night for gieing a guy a hand job (masturbation). Monday to Wednesday I made £450.' She added that it did vary quite a bit.
>
> (Red-light district)

The money itself may be an incentive to continue working as a prostitute. One consequence of this increase in cash flow is that many women find their drug habit increasing in proportion to the amount they can afford to spend on it:

> Tania said she'd earned a good bit of money the last few nights and I asked her if that meant she had money left over so she didn't have to

work every night. 'No, it's no' like that, the more money you make
the more you spend, your habit just gets bigger.'

(Red-light district)

Many women reported drug habits costing between £100 and £300 per
day. This relationship between the money available for drugs as proportio-
nate to the size of an individual drug habit has been described elsewhere
(Fields and Walters 1985). The relative speed with which women could
earn large sums of money is clear from the following field-note:

Paula (who has a heroin habit) said she was looking to make £90 so
she could get away and score before coming back out again. She and
her pal had earned £45 and £30 in the last hour. I puzzled, wasn't
heroin usually about £80 a gramme? 'Aye, it is but we need money
for taxi fares and that, fags . . . you know.'

(Red-light district)

A prostituting woman is liable to develop a heavy and expensive habit
which, in turn, may necessitate that she work longer hours and more
frequently in order to make sufficient money to pay for the drugs she needs.

Those who appeared to be under the greatest pressure were women who
were prostituting to finance their own *and* their partner's drug use:

'Many's the time I've rushed back with enough to get Bill squared up,
in the end he gave up shoplifting and stayed in his bed the whole time.
In the end I said to fuck with this, I'm away working my arse off and
he's in bed, so I said, "you're strung out now, right, so you can stay
strung out because that's me and you can find me at my Dad's", so I
left.'

(Needle exchange)

It is possible to see how once a woman begins prostituting as a solution
to the problem of funding an expensive habit she might find it difficult to
stop. The speed with which such large sums of money can be made can
serve to lock a woman further into her addiction, necessitating that she
continue prostituting to finance her drug use. It is important to recognize
this cycle of increasing drug use generating the need to work longer hours.
The pressure of this cycle may itself have a direct bearing on a woman's
ability to turn down the offer from clients of more money for unprotected
sex (Lawrinson 1991).

Some women reported the occurrence of needle and syringe sharing
between prostitutes whilst working in the city's red-light district. The red-
light district in Glasgow is based in a primarily commercial part of the city
where, at the time of the research, there were no facilities for buying or
exchanging injecting equipment. This is in stark contrast to the drug economy which is in full flow at night. Any woman working in the area and

earning enough money to buy drugs, but who does not have her own needle and syringe, will possibly have to share injecting equipment:

> We asked three women we were speaking to if they were ever asked to lend needles and syringes. 'Oh aye, like that lassie the other night goin' round askin' everyone if they'll lend her a set. She even asked me but I said I don't carry any on me. I mean she asked me and I'm a stranger. She was askin' everyone, she could've used someone's that's got AIDS.'
>
> (Red-light district)

Although there was no evidence of women working for male pimps, many of the women had males in attendance (locally known as stickmen). Most of these men were in sexual relationships with the woman they protected and were themselves injecting drug users. Similarly, some of these men were requesting the loan of injecting equipment from the women:

> As I approached a woman whom I thought to be working, a guy came over obviously intending to speak to her. I thought he was a client so I walked on by. Still within earshot I heard him ask her something about works. When he left I enquired if he'd been asking for a loan of her works. 'Aye, I gave them him'. Had she minded? 'No I dinnae mind'. Had she expected to hit up again tonight? Her answer was vague and seemed unthinking. 'Well if I can get the money together, aye'. I tried to find out if she had an extra set on her to inject but she said she had some at her house, adding 'they're shot though'.
>
> (Red-light district)

What is striking about this extract is that the woman did not see anything remarkable in passing on her needle and syringe. As we showed in Chapter 3, this is a further indication of the degree to which such passing on of equipment is integral to the sub-culture. Additionally, had the woman earned sufficient money to purchase further drugs she might well have had to borrow someone else's injecting equipment since on her own admission she had already given away her only functioning set. The risks associated with sharing within the city's red-light district may perhaps be underlined by the fact that over half of the known seropositive female drug injectors in Glasgow are known to be prostituting or to have prostituted in the recent past (Goldberg et al. 1988a).

Given the high proportion of the female prostitutes who were injecting drug users, the chances of a client contacting a female injecting drug user are very high. This likelihood would be reduced if clients were able accurately to identify which women were injecting drugs or if there were certain streets reserved for drug injecting females. Although some clients were attempting to identify which women were injecting drugs, they were not particularly successful in this regard:

One of the drug injecting prostitutes asked if we had seen a recent television programme about HIV that had had an HIV positive prostitute from Glasgow on it. The woman was quite aggrieved that the prostitute had agreed to an interview since it had reduced trade in the area. 'I've just been with a punter and he checked and double checked ma arms for track marks.' Later on that evening another drug-injecting prostitute reported that a punter had been asking her how to recognise a junkie prostitute without knowing that she was one herself.

(Red-light district)

In addition, although many of the female prostitutes did indeed describe certain streets as being reserved for non-drug injecting women, in fact many of the drug injecting women we contacted were working on streets supposedly claimed by the non-injectors.

It was pointed out by some of the non-drug injecting women that they would refuse to provide sexual services to a client whom they knew or suspected of having contacted a drug injecting prostitute:

We met Maureen and her pal, neither of whom use drugs, though Maureen says she takes a drink now and then. I asked Maureen if she ever had sex with her regulars without a condom. She said 'No never' and seemed pretty adamant. She told how recently she'd been with one of her regulars in the car and he had mentioned in passing that he had had sex with a lassie from a part of the red light district believed to be the preserve of the drug injecting women. He'd had sex without a condom. 'The tenner had been on the dash board and I'd taken it assuming it had been for me but when he said that, I said "you'd better take me back and let me outta this motor, and see you, you'd better go and get yourself a test. Those women down there are all junkies and HIV positive, well you can now fuck off and don't come to me no more".'

(Red-light district)

Given the high levels of injecting drug use we identified amongst the female prostitutes there exists the potential for spread of infection between prostitutes and their clients. The extent to which this potential is likely to be realized in practice depends on a number of factors, nearly all of which are inadequately understood at present: the extent of HIV infection among prostitutes; the relative likelihood of HIV transmission from female to male and male to female, the sort of sexual services provided by prostitutes, and finally the extent of condom use. On the latter topic we have some information.

Condom use with clients

At present the only recommended barrier against heterosexual transmission of HIV infection is the use of a condom preferably combined with spermicidal lubricant (Hearst and Hulley 1988; Stein, 1990). Although public health initiatives to encourage the use of condoms among heterosexuals have not proved entirely successful, their uptake among prostitutes is high (van den Hoek *et al.* 1989; McKeganey *et al.* 1990b). All of the women we contacted reported insisting on the use of condoms with clients. Condom use was represented as being an habitual and integral part of their work:

> Anne was describing a recent encounter with a client who had asked her to have sex without a condom. 'I don't do anythin' without a condom, I don't even do hand jobs without one.'
>
> (Red-light district)

Although the women saw condom use as part and parcel of the work, their attitude did not appear to be universally shared by their clients. This has also been found in other studies (Kinnell 1989; van den Hoek *et al.* 1989). A few of the women reported clients deliberately attempting to burst or remove condoms:

> As we were standing talking with a small group of prostitutes a woman approached saying, 'I don't know what happened to that condom but I'm feeling awful wet. I think he might have taken it off.' The others then talked about clients ripping condoms off. One of the women said 'You can always check, I always do.' The one who had approached said 'I did, I checked it was on, but I still feel awful wet.'
>
> (Red-light district)

Many of the women we spoke to reported that clients would often request sex without a condom and would be prepared to pay extra money for this service:

> We asked Sandra if she was ever asked to have sex without a condom 'you get asked every night for it without a condom, some guys'll offer £200 without one in a hotel . . . no, no they're no' usual but I mean there's not one type of guy. I mean they could be really rich or just regular kinds of guy, like just out the dancin' and wantin' a bit of business, but when you go to get the condom they're goin' "oh no, turn it up, I'm no' wearing one of them".'
>
> (Red-light district)

> Cindy says she gets asked about 3 times a week to have sex without a condom, sometimes they'll offer £100 or so, and sometimes they'll not offer anything extra.
>
> (Red-light district)

Although none of the women said that they would accept such an offer, they frequently pointed out that there were women who would provide this service. Non-drug injecting prostitutes tended to point the accusatory finger at the drug injectors:

> 'It's the junkies that's doin' it, all the junkies'. She recounted being attacked recently in a car by a guy wanting sex without a condom, 'he goes to me "your pal done me without one" I says "Ma pal? oh you must be kiddin' me on".'
>
> (Red-light district)

However, there was considerable ill-feeling between the drug injecting women and the non-drug injecting women such that one cannot accept these accusations at face value:

> We spoke to a woman who does not use drugs. She says she only comes out on Thursday and Friday of each week. She was extremely bitter about the drug users whom she says she will have little to do with. She describes them as being full of AIDS and doing business for five pounds (the going rate is ten pounds). She added that she has her regulars but that she now felt wary about taking them on because they might have been going with another woman and might pass on AIDS to her.
>
> (Red-light district)

Judging by the frequency with which reports of clients offering more money for unprotected sex were provided to us it seems highly likely, despite the universal denial of the practice, that at least some of the women were accepting such offers:

> Linda said she'd been picked up by a punter last night and when she refused to do it without a condom he said he frequently got sex without one. She replied 'if that's the case how come you've picked me up?' She added, 'he wasnae kiddin' either 'cos he pointed out the girl, knew her name and everything. He said that she'd said to him "Want to gie me something extra and I'll do it without a condom".'
>
> (Red-light district)

The tendency of the non-drug injecting women to point the finger at the drug injecting women may be no more than a feature of the underlying antagonism between the two groups. Nevertheless, drug withdrawal is an unpleasant experience reportedly and one that is alleviated by further injection. There is a strong chance then that a woman who has begun to withdraw, but who does not have sufficient money to purchase drugs may find it particularly difficult to resist the inducement of extra financial reward accompanying the request for unprotected sex:

Sally talked about experiencing withdrawal symptoms the other night;
'and there was this guy driving all round this town trying to get
someone to do it without a condom. He was offering £100 for it. It's
the first time I've ever really thought about it, you know I was like
that (she gestured to show how bad she'd felt) but I just ended up
saying "Oh no, I can't do that". In the end he got another lassie to do
it.'

(Red-light district)

Even where a woman was not experiencing withdrawal symptoms she
might still feel under a good deal of pressure to earn money, either for her
own drug habit or for her partner's, and also for other things such as
childcare, debts or court fines. Fieldwork experience suggested that even
though women who were not using drugs might also have debts to meet,
there was not the same urgency as that observed among women working to
service one or two drug habits. This was expressed by a woman who herself
injected drugs describing the difference between drug injecting prostitutes
and non-drug using prostitutes:

'A lot of junkies have got to be wider (streetwise) because the whole
time they've got a customer they're thinking about a hit and the more
money they get the more heroin they get. That's always in the mind,
how to make more money, more money.'

(Residential detoxification unit)

The situation in relation to condom use amongst the male prostitutes
seemed very much the opposite of that for the female prostitutes we contacted (Bloor et al. 1990). Whereas for the women condoms seemed an
accepted, even mundane part of their work, amongst the male prostitutes
(who tended to be in their late teens or early twenties) condoms could give
rise to some considerable embarrassment:

I asked him how many punters he had had in the last two months and
he said 2 or 3, adding that he didn't like doing it. I asked him what
services he provided and he said just wanking them off. When I asked
about condoms he laughed rather embarrassedly and said he found it
too difficult to ask for them at the chemist. I said that we had some
which we could give him if he wished and he nodded.

(Arthur Street toilets)

The male prostitute in this extract was not providing full anal sex. Nevertheless, some of the male prostitutes we contacted were providing this
service and some of them were similarly not using condoms:

Gary said that he would see on average 6 punters a day and would
often work 6 days a week. I asked him what services he would provide
and he said he got asked to let guys shag him but that he didn't like

doing that and tended to say that he would shag them. I asked about condoms and he said that he didn't carry them and only used them if the punter insisted. He did add a while later that he was concerned about the risks of HIV and I explained that unprotected anal sex was very risky and that to protect himself he ought to use a condom (at the end of our chat Mick passed him a handful of condoms under the table).

(Barkham Street toilets)

The statement that condom use was more a matter for the client to decide upon rather than the prostitute was something which many of the males expressed and which was quite the opposite for the female prostitutes we contacted.

Condom use with private sexual partners

Condoms were reported as being only rarely used by the women in their private non-commercial relationships. To understand why this was the case it is necessary to consider the part condoms played within the women's contacts with clients. For many of the women condoms were an integral feature of their work as prostitutes and as such not something which could be easily integrated into their private non-commercial relationships:

Jenna said she didn't think many women would want to use condoms with their private partners. 'I think they think to themselves, well I don't want to do it if it feels like I'm still working. I felt like that with ma boyfriend. I didnae want to use a condom . . . mostly girls that don't use condoms it's because they've got that at the back of their mind about working the town.'

(Residential detoxification unit)

To use a condom within one's private relationships was, for many of the women, to blur the distinction between work and personal life. This has similarly been reported elsewhere in Britain (Lawrinson 1991) and in the United States (Shedlin 1990). It is hardly surprising then that the majority of the female prostitutes we contacted did not use condoms with their private partners. So reluctant were the female prostitutes to use condoms in their private relationships that they might not be used even with partners who were known to be HIV positive:

I asked Harriet whether she was fearful about AIDS/HIV. She said she had began worrying about it when she was in the de-tox unit and 'People were talking about having the virus and I knew that I'd shared with people and worked in massage parlours and saunas and I started gettin' really paranoid but I had a test and it was negative.' Harriet then chatted a bit about her boyfriend, Mark, 'At first he couldnae tell me that he had the virus and we had sex without usin' a condom. He liked me so much he was frightened that if he told me I wouldn't like him. Anyway, the next day he was goin' to the hospital and I knew that must have meant that he had the virus.' I asked Harriet if the two of them now used condoms – 'No'. 'How come?' I asked. 'Well, if I was to use a condom with Mark it would be like workin' in the town and it's very important for me to keep that separate.'

(HIV counselling clinic)

The low level of condom use with private partners is in keeping with studies conducted in the Netherlands (van den Hoek *et al.* 1988) and in the United States (Cohen 1989) and elsewhere in the United Kingdom (Ward *et al.* 1990).

Where condoms were reported as being used in private non-commercial relationships the women tended to describe those occasions as being atypical, 'one off' or 'for a laugh'. The following field-notes are illustrative of the women's attitudes to condom use with their boyfriends or husbands. These appear in keeping with attitudes towards condoms voiced by heterosexuals in general:

'No, I've no need to use them. I know I've no' got the virus and I know he's no' got it, so what would be the point?'

(Red-light district)

'No, we've never used them. I could do I suppose, safer I suppose in the long run, but we don't.'

(Red-light district)

'No, I've never used condoms. A couple of times out of curiosity, y'know'. Another girl added 'once we did it for a laugh. I wouldnae though.'

(Red-light district)

Many studies have shown that drug injecting women are most likely to have partners who are also injectors, whereas the opposite is true for male injectors (Parker *et al.* 1988; Cohen *et al.* 1989; Donoghoe *et al.* 1989; McKeganey *et al.* 1989). Almost without exception the partners of drug injecting prostitute women we contacted were themselves injecting drug users. Unprotected sex with a partner who is also an injecting drug user might expose a woman to greater risk of HIV infection than that posed by clients (Rosenberg and Weiner 1988; Ward *et al.* 1990).

Condom use between the male prostitutes and their private partners also seemed relatively rare:

I asked about drugs and Gary said he didn't use any apart from Valium which was prescribed for depression. I asked him if he considered himself as gay. He thought about this for a while and said yes, he did. He said he had had a regular partner for 3 months but had recently split up with him after having discovered 'he was going behind ma back'. I asked if they had used condoms. 'Not all the time' and that this had led him to getting an AIDS test recently.

(Barkham Street toilets)

However, a few of the male prostitutes reported that they were using condoms with private partners:

I asked Tom if he had a girlfriend and he said he did but that she didn't know what he was doing. 'Sometimes she asks where I get the money from and I just say from a couple of turns (burglaries) or a couple of motors.' He said he did use condoms with his girlfriend because she was worried about getting pregnant.

(Arthur Street toilets)

The use of condoms by non-gay identified male prostitutes often seemed more for the purposes of contraception than reducing the chances of passing on to their partner any infection contracted as a result of their work as a prostitute. One of the heterosexual drug injecting male prostitutes, for example, reported not using condoms with his girlfriend because she was already pregnant.

For the female prostitutes condoms seemed to serve as a symbolic barrier differentiating between commercial and non-commercial sex. This did not appear to be as pressing a concern amongst the male prostitutes, perhaps reflecting the fact that condoms were less of a feature of the male prostitutes work. This seems to illustrate that there is considerable potential for transmission of infection between male prostitutes, their clients and their private non-commercial partners.

In the next section we will look at the relationships prostitutes establish with their clients and the ways in which these may influence the possible risk of HIV transmission between prostitutes and their clients.

Controlling the transaction

In the absence of being able to directly observe prostitute/client interactions one has to rely for information on condom use on what prostitutes say about their use. Whilst this is in some ways unsatisfactory, one can ask whether prostitutes establish the sort of relationships with clients which enable them to insist on the use of condoms. The degree to which female and male prostitutes are able to insist on condoms being used must bear some relationship to the degree to which they are in control of the interaction with clients (Shedlin 1990; Stein 1990).

Whereas in heterosexual, non-commercial relationships there is traditionally an expectation that the power balance will be weighted in favour of
the male partner (Holland *et al.* 1990b) in prostitute/client relationships it is
the female who tries to establish control. Prostitute women attempt to
create a position of some advantage based on the fact that it is they who are
selling a service to clients. From the women's accounts and also from our
own observations, it was clear that whether drug using or not, the women
sought to manage their dealings with clients. They would determine the
sexual services on offer, the price and the place where sex would be
provided. This much is clear from the following field-note:

> We stood with a group of three non-drug using prostitutes when a
> man approached on foot making a beeline for Irene. He asked her for
> sex, shaking her head she flatly replied that she didn't do sex outside.
> He then said he had a car. Looking straight at him Irene said 'well, it's
> £10 for sex in a motor'. He agreed the price and with that Irene
> walked away with him. Throughout this it was very clear that Irene
> was in control of the transaction of business, making plain her terms
> and conditions and seemingly inflexible in the application of those
> conditions.
>
> (Red-light district)

The controlling stance which the female prostitutes sought to establish with
clients did not seem similarly demonstrated by the male prostitutes. Rather, it
appeared that the client was in overall charge of the interaction, often deciding what services the male prostitute would provide, the setting where sexual
services would be provided and whether condoms would be used:

> I asked Ivan who was in charge during the contact with clients and he
> answered pretty definitely 'It's what the punter wants'. I also asked
> him if they always performed in the toilets and he said that that again
> was up to the punter.
>
> (Arthur Street toilets)

Elsewhere we have described how the relative powerlessness of many of
the male prostitutes compared to the female prostitutes may have had to do
with the fact that amongst the male prostitutes there was a convention of
only being paid *after* sexual services had been provided. Amongst the female
prostitutes it was invariably the case that the women would demand pay-
ment *prior* to providing sexual services (McKeganey *et al.* 1990b). The
important point to note here is that by adopting a controlling stance the
female prostitutes (irrespective of whether or not they inject drugs) are
much better placed to insist on condoms being used.

It is important to stress that the issue of who is in control of the interaction is itself potentially problematic since violence and intimidation seemed
an ever present feature of prostitute/client relationships:

Susan said men asked for sex without condoms frequently, 'some get aggressive if you say you don't do that'. Tanya added that earlier in the week an oldish man tried to force her into giving him oral sex without a condom. 'When I says no, he started trying to force ma head down there, so I shouted out and two lassies came down the alley and chased him'.

(Red-light district)

Another factor influencing the degree to which a woman can maintain control over the transaction relates to the quantity and type of drug she might have taken. In particular the use of the drug temazepam has been noted to be especially disinhibiting (Klee *et al.* 1990).

Many women report prostitution to be a stressful occupation; police can arrest them and clients can be dangerous. Similarly, no woman could fail to be aware of the stigma attached to the work. Women often reported that their response to these pressures was to try to numb the experience by making sure they had injected drugs both before and after work:

'Working in the streets puts a lot of pressure on your mind because of what you're doing . . . A lot of times I'd a hit before I went to ma work so I didnae think about it and then after I left ma work I'd have a hit.'

(Residential detoxification unit)

'It's no' easy money, it's quick money but it takes a lot of bottle. Your head's wasted with it, that's what used to stop me from working. I just couldnae handle it.'

(Residential detoxification unit)

The use of drugs not only as an end in itself but also to numb the experience of prostitution sometimes resulted in women working whilst clearly not in full control of themselves:

We saw Anna, a woman we know to be an injector. She staggered across the road barely able to walk and then collapsed in the doorway. Mick and I walked over to see if she had hurt herself or if she was about to overdose, she certainly looked close to it, but she pulled herself up and lurched across the road again, presumably to look for business.

(Red-light district)

It would be unfair to suggest that this is typical of all drug using prostitutes. However, the potential for this type of situation clearly exists where women who inject have adequate finance and access to drugs whilst working in an oftentimes highly stressful occupation.

Condoms and commercial sex

In the previous chapter we looked at the very low levels of condom use reported amongst drug injectors and noted that this was in keeping with low levels of reported use amongst heterosexuals as a whole. Earlier in this chapter we noted that there were low levels of condom use between female prostitutes and their private non-commercial partners. The finding that condoms are widely used in prostitute contacts with clients stands at dramatic odds with these other findings. In this section we will look at the apparent appeal of condoms for female prostitutes in their contacts with clients.

It is a commonplace to note that condoms create a physical barrier between people. Whilst such a barrier runs counter to ideas of physical and emotional closeness within private non-commercial relationships, within prostitute client contacts, by contrast, it is likely to be valued in itself. Although the latex or rubber of a condom creates only the thinnest of barriers between two people, nevertheless this may well be sufficient for the prostitute to feel that she avoids direct contact with the client. A number of anthropologists have demonstrated the symbolic value of maintaining barriers, particularly in relation to those contacts thought to be polluting of the individual or social group (Douglas 1966; Dumont 1970).

Apart from the symbolic significance of maintaining a barrier between prostitute and client, condoms are also likely to be valued for purely practical reasons. Whilst it cannot be particularly pleasant providing oral sex to someone wearing a condom, especially one that has been covered in a spermicidal lubricant, even this must be infinitely preferable to the alternative of providing oral sex without a condom to clients who vary considerably in their levels of personal hygiene.

Condoms are also likely to be appreciated for their function as a receptacle for clients' semen. Whilst the client might ejaculate within the woman, nevertheless the semen can be easily removed with the removal of the condom. This is likely to be valued for both symbolic and practical reasons especially amongst streetworking women who may have limited or no access to washroom or shower facilities.

In the previous chapter we noted that one of the reasons condoms were not being used in private relationships was because their use involved interrupting the flow of events leading to the sexual encounter. Research on gay male sexual behaviour shows a similar finding. For example Pollack et al. (1990) found that 60 per cent of their sample of gay men explained not using a condom with non-regular partners in terms of their being sexually 'turned on' at the time.

Amongst the female prostitutes, the idea of being equivalently 'turned on' with clients could hardly have been further from the reality. Sexual contacts with clients were described in unemotional terms as a matter of business. Indeed, the standard opening gambit used by nearly all of the women in their contacts with potential clients was to ask if the male was 'looking for business?' The insistence on condom use was entirely in keeping with this business-like orientation amongst the women towards sex with clients. Indeed, the insistence on condom use may have further served to underline the reality of the mechanical and unemotional nature of that sexual contact.

Condoms are valued by the female prostitutes in their dealings with clients, it seems, for the very same reasons that they are devalued by people generally in private relationships.

We turn now to look at the policy implications of our work with female and male prostitutes.

Policy and service implications

Perhaps the first point to make here is that we see no benefit whatsoever in responding to the assumed threat of HIV transmission associated with prostitution by increasing the social control of prostitutes. In addition to being ineffective in eradicating prostitution, such measures are likely to increase HIV-related risk behaviour by forcing prostitutes into increasingly covert styles of working, and out of contact with helping agencies. Recent ethnographic work on prostitute/client negotiations also supports this view (Lawrinson 1991). A concern to prevent the transmission of HIV presents a good case for the relaxation of some of the legally enforced controls on prostitution. Similarly, it is important to develop street-based agencies that have a non-threatening style of working and which are accessible to male and female prostitutes. In addition to providing condoms and sterile injecting equipment, such clinics should also provide health check-ups (particularly gynaecological services), advice on HIV risk reduction and, where necessary, referral to specialist services.

There is a particular need to encourage male prostitutes to be more directive with clients and to insist on the use of condoms. It may be valuable to provide male prostitutes with the sort of social skills training enabling them to adopt working practices similar to their female counterparts. Indeed, there may be some value in creating situations, if none already exist, where male and female prostitutes can exchange information with each other on their respective working practices.

Evidence of continuing requests from clients for unsafe sex strongly suggests the need for campaigns targeted at clients. Prostitute women have responded positively to initiatives designed to increase condom use and safer sex with clients. Such efforts need to be supported by services aimed at contacting clients, providing them with condoms and stressing the risks of unprotected sexual contact. In our own most recent work in Glasgow we have had some success at contacting clients directly within the major red-light area. Outreach work should be extended to include prostitutes *and* clients as part of a dual strategy aimed at risk reduction.

Additionally, the issue of condom use between women who prostitute and their private sexual partners should be addressed. Encouraging a greater awareness of the risks of HIV infection through unprotected sex with private partners is an important part of this process. However, attention should be paid to the significance prostitutes attach to the use of the condom as a means of distinguishing between client sexual encounters and private sexual relations. The advent of the female condom does offer the possibility of maintaining this distinction whilst at the same time protecting them against potential HIV transmission from private partners, The female condom may encourage safer sex practices between women who prostitute and their private partners though it must be added that in its present form the female condom is visually unappealing. Given the research indicating that transmission of the virus from males to females is a good deal easier than from female to male, there is an obvious case for ensuring that prostitute women have the means of protecting against HIV, not only from their clients, but also private sexual partners.

Finally, it should be noted that many of the difficulties associated with delivering any kind of service to male and female prostitutes, as well as conducting research in this area, arise as a direct result of prostitution being illegal. The question as to whether or not prostitution should be legalized has not been directly addressed here. However, it has to be said that there are few more absurd sights than the nightly drama of watching individual working women being arrested by the police, fined by the courts and returning to the streets to work longer hours to pay those fines. In the Netherlands certain cities have experimented with the practice of legalizing prostitution in particular streets and providing well lit car parks with screened off sections where the women can take clients (Kleinegris 1991). Such an approach makes it easier to deliver health services to the women and reduces the likelihood of their being attacked by clients. It is debatable whether or not there is the political will in the United Kingdom to adopt similar approaches. However, there must surely be better ways of responding to prostitution, particularly in the light of AIDS, than enforced legal controls which, far from removing prostitution, serve to drive it further underground.

══ Chapter 6 ══

Living with the virus: drug injectors' experiences of HIV

Introduction

There is a growing body of literature reporting on the experience of being HIV positive, of living with the many opportunistic infections associated with ARC and AIDS and, in some cases of facing one's own imminent death (McMullen 1988; Callen 1989; Cruz 1989; Dreuilhe 1989; Sandsrom 1990; McCann and Wadsworth 1991; Siegel and Krauss 1991). In the main these accounts have either been provided by, or focused upon, male homosexuals, and as a result we know much less about the comparable experiences of drug injectors, women, haemophiliacs and young children. In this chapter we describe the experience of those drug injectors we contacted who had already been diagnosed as HIV positive. We look at their reactions to hearing the news of being positive, of communicating the diagnosis to others and the impact of being HIV positive on their relationships. We also look at how these men and women viewed the future.

The experience of HIV infection, however, is in no way confined solely to those individuals who are already living with the virus. AIDS and HIV also have an impact in one way or another on the lives of all those who see themselves as possibly at risk. We will therefore start this chapter by looking at the perceptions and reactions of drug injectors generally to the threat of HIV and AIDS.

Attitudes towards the virus

It is impossible to overstate the sense of fear which AIDS and HIV generated amongst the overwhelming majority of drug injectors we contacted. Many people described themselves as feeling 'paranoid' at anything having to do with the subject:

I asked him if he was worried about AIDS. He replied 'In truth I am. Every time I'm taking a hit I'm paranoid.' I asked him if the fear of being HIV positive had encouraged him to seek treatment. He said it had.

(Hospital detoxification ward)

Gail chatted about how she got into drugs as a result of people she was hanging around with. I asked her if she was concerned about AIDS/ HIV. 'Oh, I'm dead paranoid. See I know people who have the virus and they're not looking at all good. They're continuing to hit up.' I asked Gail what she thought would happen to people who had the virus 'I think most of them are going to get full blown AIDS.' Gail added that if she herself got the virus she would stop using drugs altogether.

(HIV counselling clinic)

Such feelings led some people deliberately to avoid any information relating to AIDS and HIV:

When I asked him initially if he was afraid of AIDS he said no, he didn't care, in fact he'd be glad if he did get it because he was so sick of living. Later on he said 'I don't know why I said I'm not afraid, I am afraid, I wouldn't know what to do with myself if I got it.' He says he never talks about it and always switches off the television when they start talking about it. I asked him if he knew anyone who was HIV positive. 'Aye, Tommy'. He's in the hospital at the moment. They met at a local drug detoxification unit – 'We were both in a bad way because we'd just split up with our girlfriends so we stuck together and helped each other.' He went on to say how terrible it must be for him and how sick he looks. I said I thought he looked okay. 'No, you should have seen him in the detox unit, a big muscley fella and now he's so thin.'

(Hospital detoxification unit)

For some people their fear of AIDS and HIV had led them to avoid even discussing the disease with friends and family:

I asked Garry whether people he knew talked about AIDS. 'No, it's a black subject. There's some people who still believe you cannae catch it.' We then talked about having the virus and Garry said that he thought you could have it and be a carrier for life without necessarily going on to develop AIDS.

(HIV counselling clinic)

Although such feelings were expressed by many people it would be a mistake to assume that all of the drug injectors we spoke to were equally concerned about the virus. A few people seemed more concerned at the possible risks of hepatitis than HIV, concentrating first and foremost it seemed on the physical signs of illness:

> I asked if he'd been in a situation recently when he'd shared his works. 'Aye, two months ago.' When I asked him to describe the situation he just said 'You don't think about it, you just do it.' He later made it clear that what he meant was he'd lent his works out, not shared them – 'but I have used other people's before, not now though, not since I've been coming here.' It didn't seem to be a fear of AIDS that made him start being careful with needles. He said he wasn't bothered about it. 'It's not something I really think about. I just saw ma pal and he got hep and then I didn't want to share ma works.' Marina: 'So it wasn't a fear of AIDS so much as a fear of hep?' 'Aye, you could see it, his face all yellow.' He seemed to be responding to the physical expression of illness.
>
> (Needle exchange)

One or two people expressed the view that AIDS and HIV perhaps offered a way of ending their life. When said in the company of others such feelings would often draw a shocked response:

> Terry (drug injecting prostitute) asked Elaine (nurse) if it was true that to get detox in the city you had to have the virus. Elaine explained that that wasn't the case. The girl then responded that she hoped she had the virus. One of the older prostitutes responded in horror at this 'You wish you had the virus. I've never heard anything like that.' After the prostitute who had said she hoped she had the virus left, Elaine said that some people say things for effect, to which the elder prostitute responded 'Yes, but she was saying things like that in the jail.'
>
> (Prostitute drop-in centre)

Amongst many of the drug injectors there was a widespread pessimism as to the likely outcome of becoming infected:

> I asked Malcolm if he ever talked about AIDS and HIV with his friends. 'Not now, I used to like but not now. Anyway a lot of ma friends have the virus.' I asked how they were keeping. 'One of them looks pretty rough but the others are alright.' Malcolm added though that he thought all of them would go on to develop AIDS and die.
>
> (HIV counselling clinic)

While most people seemed to have an accurate knowledge of how the virus was transmitted, their attitudes also seemed to have been shaped in part by possibly apocryphal stories of deliberate revenge infection:

> I asked him if he was concerned about AIDS and HIV. 'When I first heard about it I was, but I never share my tools and I never lend them

out so I dinnae think I'll get it. I might have it. I don't know. I've not been tested but if I did have it I'd never lend out my tools to anyone but I know plenty of folk who've got it and think if I've got it some other bastard is goin' to get it same as me.'

(Pharmacy)

It is important to stress that none of the individuals diagnosed as HIV positive to whom we spoke described themselves as ever having deliberately spread infection. Although it is not possible entirely to rule out revenge infection it is worth noting that similar stories were reported by Defoe in 1722 in his *Journal of the Plague Years*:

> The citizens pressing to be received and harboured in times of distress, and with the plague upon them, complain of the cruelty and injustice of the country people in being refused entrance and forced back again with their goods and families; and the inhabitants, finding themselves so imposed upon, and the citizens breaking in as it were upon them whether they would or no, complain that when they were infected they were not only regardless of others, but even willing to infect them; neither of which was really – that is to say in the colours they were described in.

(Defoe 1986: 168)

It seems highly likely that stories of revenge infection flourish in situations in which there are deep divisions and suspicions between different people and different social groups. It might be thought that such suspicions would be less likely between drug injectors, who undoubtedly had a shared culture; nevertheless it was clear from our interviews that being HIV positive could create an enormous gulf between people who might otherwise have much in common.

Since many of the fears drug injectors expressed about HIV crystallized around the issue of HIV testing it will be worthwhile looking at their experiences in this area.

HIV testing

Very many of the drug injectors we contacted reported having been tested for HIV. The greatest proportion of these reported being tested not because of their own concerns as to whether or not they were infected, but as a result of other people's concern over their injecting drug use. Quite a few people, for example, reported being tested in hospital before undergoing a clinical procedure, others reported having been tested whilst undergoing drug detoxification:

Arthur has been on the ward for 2 days. He seemed really drowsy, also he said he was depressed and wanting to leave the ward. He didn't want to though because he wanted to prove his Ma wrong. Talking to him was not particularly easy because he seemed so sleepy and also irritable. He also kept casting me in the role of counsellor and was particularly anxious to know about HIV/AIDS, its history, its spread and its relation to him. He's just agreed to have the test which may explain his preoccupation with it. He said he thought they would all think he had the virus if he refused to get the test. 'The staff asked me if I wanted to take the test. I said "Give me a bit of time. I'm only just in the door" but then all the others in here have had it and I feel left out of it so I went to the Nurse and said to put me down for the AIDS test.'

(Hospital detoxification unit)

It was clear that some drug injectors had experienced a good deal of pressure from medical staff to be tested for HIV:

Jackie described how on entering the drug detoxification unit she had been told by one of the doctors that she would have to be tested for HIV. Although her friend had agreed to be tested she had been reluctant to do so. She said that the doctor had not mentioned the question of HIV testing again.

(Hospital detoxification unit)

Some individuals reported having been tested whilst in prison:

I asked her about when she found out she had the virus. 'I was in jail and they just called me in and said I had AIDS. I couldn't speak afterwards and just went back to ma cell.' I asked Michelle if she had any idea when she might have picked up the virus. 'Aye, I know when it was, it was when I was with Sally and Sharon and Sally had made up the stuff. I said "Alright then, where's mine?" and she said "It's in the tools there". I said "What do you mean, you know I don't hit up" and she said "Well you'll have to this time because that's all there is". I'd never hit up before and I had an AIDS test before, when I had ma child which was negative so I know when it was.' I asked Michelle if she still saw Sally. 'I see her sometimes – yes, to say hello. We're not really friends, but I don't hold it against her because she didn't know she had the virus.'

(HIV clinic)

The pressure to be tested was also described as arising from non-injecting family members:

I asked her if she'd not been worried at this time by AIDS/HIV publicity – 'No, not really. Like when it came on the telly I just thought, "Oh, that shite". I never thought it had anything to do with me.' I wondered what had led Kay to come up for an AIDS test – 'My Ma was gettin' on at me and I was worryin' that if I had anythin' I might pass it on to others so I thought I might as well find out.' I asked Kay if she had thought about what she would do if it was a positive result. She laughed, obviously a bit embarrassed and said 'I'd take an overdose and finish it.'

(HIV counselling clinic)

Some individuals felt that they ought to be tested not so much as a result of the concern of other family members, but as a result of their concern for their own children:

I spoke to Paul just prior to the doctor taking his blood sample. He described himself as hitting up continuously for 7 years – 'Like I think I'm addicted to the needle since I get nothin' off it now at all.' I asked him why he had decided to get tested just now. 'Well, ma girlfriend got an appointment and I said "Well there's not a lot of use just one of us gettin' tested" so I said I'd come along too. We wouldnae have come up but for the wean. It's for his sake that we decided to get tested. If it had only been for us we wouldnae have bothered.'

(HIV counselling clinic)

It was clear that there was considerable scope for confusion surrounding the whole issue of HIV testing. Some individuals, for example, believed themselves to be HIV negative on the basis of a previous test result even though they had subsequently shared needles or had unprotected sex. Others believed themselves to be HIV negative on the basis not of their own test result, but that of another person with whom they had shared injecting equipment or had unprotected sex:

I asked him if he was worried about AIDS. 'Aye, I am.' He added that he knew he didn't have AIDS because he had shared with his brother who 3 months later had a negative AIDS test, 'so that proves that I've not got it.'

(Needle exchange)

The issue of HIV testing was enormously significant for many of the drug injectors we contacted. This was so even if this significance had been largely imposed on them as a result of other people's concern over their injecting drug use. There is cause for concern, however, in the suggestion that some individuals were being pressured into being tested. It is largely irrelevant whether such pressure is exerted alongside the offer of pre- and post-test counselling since at present, at least, we do not have information on the effectiveness of counselling in this area.

Reactions to the news of being positive

We spoke to some people who were awaiting a test result and it was clear that this was a period of almost unparalleled anxiety:

His opening gambit was how nervous he feels about the forthcoming result from his HIV test. 'I'm no' sleepin' or nothin' and I'm dreamin' of HIV clinics. I feel like I'm gonnae collapse, you know, like I'm gonnae faint. I just can't seem to get it out of my mind.' The test results are out in two days.

(Needle exchange)

The reactions to hearing the news of being positive were similarly described in terms of shock, disbelief and of time standing still:

'When I was in the rehabilitation unit I got the test to assure myself that I was negative and things didn't exactly work out that way. I remember after being told I had it I went back to my room and I was just numb. I sat there lookin' at the wall for one, two hours. It was the only time in my life I've been totally unaware of time passing. It was like I had a safety valve in ma head that said "this is too heavy so I'm shuttin down completely".'

(HIV clinic)

For many people the news of being HIV positive meant only one thing – that they were going to die in the near future:

Michelle became rather quiet and seemed to withdraw into herself. After a while she spoke very quietly and said she couldn't believe that she had the virus. 'I know I've got it. I knew I had it even before I was told. I just knew it. When they told me I thought Oh ma God ah'm gonnae be dead in two months.'

(HIV clinic)

Jane described how she had found out she had the virus. 'I was due in for an operation on ma liver and the doctor asked if he could check for HIV. I didnae really know what that was and when they called me back they said they got the results of ma HIV and hepatitis tests and one of them was positive and it wasnae ma hepatitis. I remember I just wanted to get out of there and go to ma sister's house. I thought I was dyin' and I didnae hear another word they said. When I came back later though Dr Thomas explained everything to me'.

(HIV clinic)

There is nothing unusual in these reactions; indeed, one might anticipate similar reactions from any individual being told that he or she has a life-threatening disease. However, where a person was tested as a result of someone else's concern at the fact of their injecting drug use then it seems likely that being provided with a positive test result would be even more of a shock:

> I asked him how he felt about being positive. 'I still cannae really accept it. Y'know some days I just cannae believe I've got it.' I asked him how he had found out. 'I came in here to come off and they asked me if I wanted the test. I'd had it a couple of times before when I was in the jail and they'd come back negative, so I said "Aye, nae bother". Then the test came back positive and I was shattered. You see I was not one for sharing needles.' I asked him about counselling, if it helped. 'No, it's no help. They cannae help you. I mean they say you'll be alright and that, but you can only really talk to someone that's got it as well'. He then added that most of his friends also had the virus but that they all avoided talking about it pretending it hadn't happened. 'Everyone's scared they're goin' to die tomorrow.'
>
> (Hospital detoxification unit)

It is not possible to say with any certainty that an individual's ability to cope is influenced by the situation in which a positive test result is communicated to them. Nevertheless, our data did indicate that being diagnosed as HIV antibody positive could lead to a short-term increase in risk behaviour:

> Stuart (unprompted by me), said that he had found out about his HIV when he was in London. 'I'd gone to the hospital for a test and it came back positive. I was really shocked and I think I had a sort of breakdown because from using recreationally I started usin' all the time, stayin' up for days on end and then crashing out.'
>
> (HIV counselling clinic)

Once the initial shock and disbelief of being positive had subsided it seemed a common practice for individuals to try to work out in their own minds the time and place in which they might have contracted the virus. In almost all of the cases, the situations described involved needle sharing rather than possible sexual transmission:

> I then asked Shona if she ever thought about when she got the virus. 'I think it was after I'd met this lassie in London and me and a friend went over to Edinburgh to see her. I'd not taken ma tools over wi' me and this lad called round to see her when we were there. He hit up, then she did and then I did, and then he said that he had the virus. I said, "God, why didn't you tell me?" and he just said that he thought we all knew. I was sick after that.'
>
> (HIV counselling clinic)

He says he's been using for the past 6/7 years and is now 34. Both he and his girlfriend are HIV positive. 'I think I know how it happened. I had one box for dirty needles and one for clean. One time some of my pals came round and they used the clean ones but left them in the wrong box. That's the only way it could've happened 'cos I never share ma works.' He used to get his needles from a friend who worked in the hospital and could supply him with the big boxes of used syringes. He said he'd known his diagnosis before he was tested and formally found positive.

(Hospital detoxification unit)

One of the most striking features about some of these stories was the way in which such speculations would not necessarily jeopardize the relationships between the various people involved:

Mike stated at the outset of our interview that he was HIV positive that he had never attempted to hide the fact from other people. He went on to explain that he knew the boy that had passed the virus onto him 'He knew he had the virus when he let me use his works but he's ma best friend and I can't hate him for that.' Mike explained that the boy was still his best friend even though he now has full blown AIDS. At this point Mike turned to his girlfriend and said 'What was I like when I saw him? I was greetin' and I hugged him, he's ma best mate.'

(Pharmacy)

It was also clear, however, that such suspicions could form the basis of deep-seated and long-standing resentments:

Lesley described the circumstances in which she felt she had contracted the virus. 'I was with this lassie from Charleston who I heard had the virus but I did'nae believe it. Anyway, she said we could hit in her house since she had a set of tools, so we did and it was only three weeks after that I was tested positive. The next time I saw her I wanted to kill her but she said she had only found out herself but I said "you're a lyin bastard".'

(HIV clinic)

Communicating the diagnosis to others

Deciding whom to communicate the information of being positive, as well as deciding how to avoid communicating the diagnosis to others, posed enormous problems for many of the HIV positive injectors we interviewed. Such issues were raised not on a once and for all basis, but recurrently throughout everyday life as they sought to negotiate the issue of disclosure in a multitude of different and sometimes overlapping situations and relationships.

Some of the individuals to whom we spoke had decided to keep the fact of being HIV positive a secret from as many people as possible:

> Cindy described how she had decided not to tell people about having the virus. 'Like the way I look at it is that I've got it but I don't want people feeling sorry for me or avoiding me because of it.'
>
> (HIV clinic)

On occasion such secrecy could include the individual's sexual partner:

> I asked Irene if she had a boyfriend at the moment 'Aye he doesnae know I'm HIV positive. We're just engaged. I think he might guess since we're using condoms. Well, I say we're using condoms but we've no had sex for months because ma head's so done in.'
>
> (HIV clinic)

Keeping such a momentous secret to oneself was far from easy. As the extract above well illustrates, even amongst those who had opted for this strategy there was a feeling that their sexual partner might have begun to suspect the truth behind their evasions.

A few individuals seemed to have opted for the opposite strategy, of being as open as possible about the fact of having the virus:

> Immediately into our conversation Thomas starts off by saying that he is HIV positive, adding that he supposed I knew that already. I said that I did not and he said 'Well I have not hidden it from anybody, all my friends know.'
>
> (HIV clinic)

More common than either of these strategies, however, was the approach of confiding in a small number of close friends or relatives:

> I asked Kathy if she felt able to tell people about having the virus. 'Yes' she said 'ma family have been very good and so has ma boyfriend's family.' Her boyfriend she said was an ex-junkie. 'He thinks he's got the virus but he'll no' get checked, and when we have sex we always use a Durex.' Kathy obviously felt really supported in this relationship saying that they were soon to move to Ireland where they were going to try and set up a new life for themselves.
>
> (HIV clinic)

> Jack said that only two people, his sister and his brother-in-law, knew that he had the virus. 'I don't talk about it and I think that those that do are really daft since you never know how people are going to react to it'.
>
> (HIV clinic)

Although this strategy opened up the possibility of being able to benefit from the comfort and support of selected others, it also involved relinquishing a measure of control over further disclosures:

> In the bedroom Clive gave his version of the story. He'd been up at his mother's and when he came in Jane had said to him that Mikey (her brother) might mention the virus to him. 'I thought what's he wantin' to talk about the virus just like that for, she must have told him. Anyway, so I go into the sitting room and Jane says to Mikey "I think Clive's got somethin' he wants to tell you" so then I'm lookin' like a stupid cunt.' He then turned to Jane and said she'd really hurt him by telling Mikey herself and not letting him do it. Jane justified this saying 'I know my brother. I know what he's like. He jumps about with Tom and other people in Parkland. I didn't want him to find out from one of them when it should come from me. I'm his family aren't I? He should hear it from me first.' Clive said he wanted to tell the guy but Jane had kept saying 'no, no, don't tell him, he'll go nuts'. As part of the effort to calm down the situation Jane said that Mikey thought he had the virus anyway.
>
> (Streetwork field-note)

There were two areas where individuals found themselves repeatedly negotiating their way around the issue of informing others; one was in relation to requests to share injecting equipment and the other was in relation to possible sexual contacts.

Drug use and needle sharing

Most of the HIV positive drug injectors we interviewed were continuing to inject. Only four people said that they had stopped using drugs as a result of becoming HIV positive. One person said that she had switched from injecting to snorting drugs as a result of being positive. Some of those who were continuing to inject explained this in terms of their HIV positive diagnosis. A few people, for example, found themselves using increasing amounts of their chosen drug as a way of coping with psychological stress:

> I asked her if she felt her sense of the future was different now that she knew she had the virus. 'Everything is different. I get really depressed about things and I think about killing myself. I don't think the doctors really understand what it's like. I don't think anybody understands who hasn't got it. When I do get depressed I think more and more about smack. I'm dabbling now, but I know if it goes on like this I'll be addicted.'
>
> (HIV clinic)

I asked Tommy if he filtered his smack 'No, it's a fuckin waste there's so much rubbish in it if you start filterin it you'll get nothin' of it.' Tommy then reiterated that he had to come off drugs altogether or his girlfriend was going to start using again, however he also added 'Mind you what's the point when I know I've got the virus and I'm gonna be dead anyway. I might as well take all I can get.'

(HIV clinic)

By no means all of the drug users, however, were as pessimistic in their view of the future as the man in the extract above. A few people, for example, were attempting to reduce their drug use because of their diagnosis as HIV positive:

I asked him about any current drug use and he said that the last time he had had a hit was two weeks ago. 'I'm not saying I'm off it because if somebody offered it I'd take it but I'm not taking it all the time.' He explained to me that the stuff speed and smack are cut with can attack your T4 cells, 'so I know that it is better if I was off it altogether.'

(HIV clinic)

It would be wrong though to explain these individuals' continued drug use solely in terms of their being positive. Of at least equal weight was the fact that nearly all of them continued to live in areas where there was little opportunity of finding employment, where drug injecting was widespread and where most of their friends were also injecting:

Patrick talked at length about his craving for Tems saying that he had recently hit up and adding that his girlfriend gets on at him for it 'But when I see all of ma pals full of it I have this jealousy inside me'. He reiterated that his girlfriend did not understand the nature of his craving and complained that when his mates came up for him that she would shout at them. I asked him if he did not feel that she was doing this with his best interests at heart. 'No,' he said 'I need ma pals around me. I've grown up with them.'

(HIV clinic)

We have already noted in Chapter 3 that some of the HIV positive drug injectors had been asked to pass on their injecting equipment to others. Such requests raised the possibility of having to inform the person that they were HIV positive. For some individuals, this did not seem to pose any great difficulty:

Jenny said that she had never made a secret of the fact of having the virus. 'At first people used to say "can I have a lend of your works" and I'd say I had the virus and they'd back off. Now it's not so bad.'

(HIV clinic)

However, for those people who were not so open about being positive such requests could present considerable difficulties. To avoid those problems some individuals sought to avoid injecting in the company of others:

> I asked Paula whether she was currently using. 'Yes I get through a gramme a day' I asked if she injected 'No I snort it. I'm always with other people when I use and they're always chapping me for a loan of ma tools and I know that I'd have to tell them they couldnae use them because I had the virus.'
>
> (HIV clinic)

Some others sought to turn down requests to share injecting equipment, not by explaining that they were HIV positive, but by commenting that the person requesting the injecting equipment might be:

> I asked Shona about lending equipment. 'There's no way I'd do it. I wouldn't wish this on ma worst enemy. I've been asked for ma works but I just say no and they'll say how can you no help me I'm pure strung out, and I'll say "look I've no got the virus but I don't know about you so I'm no sharin ma tools".'
>
> (HIV clinic)

We have already noted that none of the HIV positive drug injectors we interviewed reported deliberately sharing injecting equipment out of a conscious attempt to spread the virus. Indeed, all of the seropositives were acutely aware of the risks they posed to others. Some people did, however, describe situations in which they had either used other people's injecting equipment or had their equipment used by others.

A few people felt that when asked to pass on their injecting equipment it was sufficient to tell the person that they were positive, leaving it up to them to decide whether or not to borrow the injecting equipment:

> I asked Rachel if people asked her for a loan of her tools 'This fella came up to me yesterday for a loan and I said "I have a clean barrel but I don't have a spike" so he said "just give me what you've got and I'll boil it." I said "take what you like but you're not hittin' up in ma house because you'll be tellin' people you got the virus from me".' I asked Rachel if she had told the guy that she had the virus. 'Yes I tell everybody. I think I should tell people about it and if they want to talk about it it's their affair. There's been one or two that's been difficult.'
>
> (HIV clinic)

Other individuals described situations in which someone else had used their injecting equipment:

> Gail said that there were lots of people still sharing in the part of Glasgow in which she lived. 'Sometimes at night and at the weekend you can't get a set of tools. Like the other day I was full of it and so

> was ma boyfriend's brother and he wanted a shot of ma tools and I said you'll have to boil them but he wasnae bothered'.
>
> (HIV clinic)

It would clearly be quite wrong to describe such situations in terms of revenge infection.

There were also reports of group sharing involving a seropositive drug injector, we described one such occasion in the chapter on needle sharing:

> I asked Lesley about needle sharing and she said it was happening regularly still. I asked her to describe a recent situation – 'There was a group of eight of us in this guy's house with one set of tools. They knew I was positive so they used the one set and left me till last.'
>
> (HIV clinic)

On this occasion the individual was clearly attempting to reduce the risk she posed to others.

Relationships with others

Most of the seropositive drug injectors we interviewed felt extremely pessimistic about the possibility of forming any long-term meaningful sexual relationship with others. Forming such relationships meant having to communicate their HIV diagnosis, and that, for many, was too difficult to face:

> I asked her if she could see herself getting involved with a guy. 'If I did get involved I would tell him from the start that I had the virus, but to be honest I'm no' interested now in all that because I've worked in the town (prostitution) but also because I don't think there's too many guys who would want to get involved with someone who had the virus.'
>
> (HIV clinic)

Sylvia talked at length about how things have changed for her now that she knew about the virus. 'I don't go out to the dancin' or the discos. There's no point in me meeting a guy now and ma family react different to me.' In what way I asked? 'I dunno, just different.'

(HIV clinic)

Simon said that he felt he would quite like a boyfriend but that at the moment all he had were one night stands. Simon added a while later that he would never tell these people about his HIV but was well aware of the difficulties if the relationship did become long-term.

(HIV clinic)

A few of the HIV positive men and women seemed more optimistic about the possibility of establishing or maintaining longer term relationships. Some people had adopted a strategy of informing a prospective partner at the earliest possible point about being HIV positive:

Stevie spoke at length about girls. 'I have a girlfriend at the moment who I have been seeing for 2 years. She knows I have the virus. I tell everybody. I think it's better that they know at the outset because I couldnae handle telling someone, say, 10 minutes before going to bed with them. If you don't tell them at the beginning when do you tell them? after the first week or month? You can't do that. They have a right to know.'

(HIV clinic)

While it was evident that being HIV positive could exert an intolerable strain on relationships some people described instances in which being positive had led to a rapprochement in certain relationships. In the main though this seemed to be the case with family members rather than sexual partners:

I asked Sally if she hit up now and she said no adding that she thought HIV had helped her. 'HIV has bought a lot of positive things. I know that sounds pretty strange but it has, like ma Da and me are really close. We talk about who's going to die first and what sort of funeral we'll have.'

(HIV clinic)

Amongst others, however, the stresses produced by having a family member who was both drug injector and HIV positive could strain family relationships to breaking point:

Rachel then talked a bit about her family. 'I have a younger brother and an older sister. Ma brother hates me and I hardly see ma sister. When ma Da found out I had the virus it nearly killed him. He came up to the hospital to see Dr Graham saying he would pay anything to get me into a clinic to get rid of the virus but Dr Graham explained to him that I was not dying, but now we don't even speak to each other since we fell out.' I asked Rachel where she was staying now and she said that though she had her own flat she was staying with her Aunt.

(HIV clinic)

As well as undermining hopes for the formation of long-term sexual relationships in the future, for some people the fact of being positive had also undermined existing relationships:

Linnie talked a bit about sexual matters. She said that she'd had a boyfriend who had wanted to keep seeing her. 'But I kept thinking I

wouldnae want to pass it on to him or his wee girl and anyway he was
seeing another woman who was tellin' him he shouldnae be seein'
me.' I asked her if she felt she would meet someone else and she said
'no, I couldnae face havin' to tell a guy I had the virus.' What about
one night stands I asked, 'couldn't you imagine not telling the guy and
using a condom?' 'No', she said, 'I'm no' one for one night stands, I'm
too shy.'

(HIV clinic)

In Chapter 4 we looked at the difficulties of using condoms within the
context of long-term relationships. These difficulties were experienced
even more acutely by seropositive men and women who were involved in
long-term relationships:

I had earlier asked Gail about wearing condoms and she returned to
this saying that she couldn't all the time be finding excuses for wearing
a condom but nor could she consider not wearing one. 'Ma boyfriend
would like to have sex without one but I couldn't face passing this on
to anyone else.' She fell silent for a while then said 'what man's gonnae
want to wear a condom all the time? – what do you call it, like havin'
a bath with your socks on.' I had laughed when I heard this phrase
before but now it made me feel incredibly sad. My protestations that if
a guy liked someone enough he would be prepared to wear condoms
seemed empty even to me.

(HIV clinic)

For some of those people who were in long-term relationships there was a
feeling that since they had not been using condoms before being told that
they were HIV positive, there was little point in using them after the
diagnosis:

Clare said that her boyfriend knew about her being positive and added
that he refused to get tested. 'He says if he hasn't got it now he won't
get it and if he has got it he does not want to know.' I asked if they
were using condoms. 'No we've been together for three years now so
what's the point in startin' to use them now?'

(HIV clinic)

It is now known that people who are HIV positive are infectious to
differing degrees at different points during the course of their illness. The
fact that one might not have been using condoms in the past does not mean
that there is little point in wearing them after learning of an HIV positive
diagnosis. However, one can see how this belief might exist within the
context of a long-term relationship.

In discussing the difficulties of establishing or maintaining long-term
relationships, the topic of children was always near to the surface. At the

time at which this study was carried out many of the seropositive injectors had been actively counselled against having children. Having to remain childless was frequently cited as the worst aspect of being positive. It was this topic more than any other, including that of facing possible death from the disease, which gave rise to the most emotional upset in our interviews. This was true for both the women and the men we spoke to:

> I asked Terry if there were times when he felt really low and he said not really, but that he did feel sad at the knowledge he would not have a family. 'I couldnae do that, I couldnae bury a coffin a foot long. I would have liked a child, a son who I could have taken to football and that, but I know the risks outweigh the pleasure I would get. Anyway ma brother has a daughter and I'm kind of a father figure to her so there's children in ma life.'
>
> (HIV clinic)

> The last thing Sally and I spoke about was children, with Sally saying that the worst thing about having the virus was not being able to have children – 'I love children, I always have, and now I know I can never have any that's the hardest part.'
>
> (HIV clinic)

> Jenny talked a bit about her boyfriend saying that he had been really helpful when he had found out about her being positive and that he had wanted them to stay together. I asked her if they were using condoms and she said that he was in the gaol just now. She then spoke about not being able to have children 'I told him that sooner or later he was gonnae want children and that I was not gonnae be able to have any'. Jenny became quite weepy at this point and asked me what advice I would give her about starting a family. I explained that the best person she should discuss that with was the doctors she would be seeing in a short while.
>
> (HIV clinic)

Some of the HIV positive females had been informed of being positive as a result of an HIV test carried out during their pregnancy. Where this had happened it had led to some individuals being counselled against continuing with the pregnancy:

> Irene talked a bit about the effects of heroin. I asked her whether at the time she was injecting she knew anything about HIV. 'Not really. I only found out about it because I got pregnant. I was really thin when I was on smack and then when I came off I put on a lot of weight and ma boyfriend said to me one day that I looked pregnant. I hadn't had a period for ages and I didn't think there was any chance I could have been pregnant but when I got tested they told me I was

twenty weeks. I was also tested for HIV and when they told me I was positive and explained all the figures to me I made my mind up that there was no way I was gonnae bring a wean into the world with AIDS so I just said I'd have an abortion.'

(HIV clinic)

What further underscores the obvious upset created by deciding against continuing with pregnancy on this basis is that at the time of writing the most recent estimate of the likelihood of a mother passing on infection to an unborn child is 13 per cent (European Collaborative Study 1991). This is considerably lower than the previous estimates on which some of these women would have based their decision to remain childless or to terminate a pregnancy. Similarly, the belief that pregnancy itself may hasten the development of illness in an HIV positive female is no longer held to be the case. Given the current state of knowledge about transmission of the virus from a mother to her baby there seems little reason why an HIV positive woman should not feel she can have a child if that is what she wishes.

Perceptions of the future

In discussing what the future might hold for each of these individuals one could have been enquiring about any number of topics; in reality, of course, there was one topic which overrode all others, namely the possibility of progressing to ARC and AIDS, and of dying prematurely. As with virtually every aspect of the reality of being positive there were enormous differences in the ways in which the future was regarded. Some people seemed to have almost an unshakeable faith in their capacity to remain well:

Sylvia described herself as being optimistic. 'I don't think I'm going to die for another 30 years or so unless I get run over by a car, but that's the way I am.' Sylvia contrasted this with her boyfriend who is also HIV positive by saying that he thought he would be dead in 6 months and if not then, within a year. 'He has really dark moods like he always used to have a temper on him and once a week he'd have a good shouting but now he doesnae shout. He just gets really moody. Like if I see anything in the paper on AIDS or on television, I want to see it but he just screws it up or switches it off. He puts on a happy face when he's outside but I see him at home and at night when he is going to sleep. He goes really rigid and talks in his sleep, "please don't let me die".'

(HIV clinic)

Others though were beginning to draw distinctions between the quality of their life and how long it might last which suggested that they were coming to accept the possibility of their own premature death:

> Simon described how he felt sure that he wasn't going to get AIDS. 'I eat brown bread and yoghourt and keep myself relatively fit.' A while later Simon emphasised that he felt what was important was not so much the length of one's life but its quality.
>
> (HIV clinic)

Still others seemed to hold a very pessimistic view of what the future might hold. Five of the 26 seropositive individuals we interviewed, for example, drew explicit attention to their preparedness to commit suicide in the face of a transition from being HIV positive to ARC and AIDS:

> I asked her if she felt her sense of the future was different now that she knew she had the virus. 'Everything is different. I get really depressed about things and I think about killing myself.'
>
> (HIV clinic)

> Marion lapsed into silence again which I didn't really want to interrupt. I was going to ask her about her recent holiday when she suddenly stated 'If I get full blown AIDS I'm no gonnae lie and die in a hospital bed' She began to cry. 'I'll do what I did last time when I was depressed – I'll take an overdose.' I asked her what had got her so depressed. She wiped the make-up from her eyes and I told her that if it upset her we didn't have to talk. 'No I want to. It's just that it sets me off greetin'. There was lots of things that were upsettin' me knowin' that I couldnae have a family which I wanted and knowin' that I would never settle down with a man.'
>
> (HIV clinic)

Such sentiments were even expressed on occasion by individuals who otherwise seemed fairly optimistic about their capacity to remain well.

It is noteworthy in this regard that mortality amongst a group of drug injectors in Edinburgh showed increasing deaths by overdose, particularly by individuals who were HIV positive and female. Whilst it is not always clear whether death by overdose is accidental or intentional, the researchers suggest that some of these overdoses might have been suicides (Skidmore *et al.* 1990). Given the anxiety and trauma which many of the HIV positive men and women in this study reported experiencing, it is not difficult to see how suicide might come to be seen as one way of dealing with their situation.

> I asked Michelle if she thought much about the virus. 'I do sometimes. Like I think there's no way I'm goin' to lie and die in hospital with full blown AIDS. I'd kill myself before it got to that.' Michelle then said that she felt she should try and keep herself well. I asked her what she meant by that and she said by not injecting. I asked her if she had

stopped and she said she had but that she had had two recent hits when her methadone had been stolen.

(HIV counselling clinic)

Among those men and women who spoke about committing suicide it was noticeable that their recurrent fear was of themselves dying alone in a hospital bed. This is an image that has been portrayed many times in media representations of AIDS.

It was a disappointing feature of our interviews that so few of the HIV positive injectors regarded themselves as having any control over their own health. A few individuals made reference to minor changes they had made to their diet and a few others spoke generally about trying to 'keep themselves well' as a way of attempting to reduce the likelihood of disease progression:

> Sally commented that she took more care of herself now as a result of having the virus, 'Like if someone has a cold I'm careful not to get too close, also I go for walks and things like that'.

(HIV clinic)

Although only a few people saw themselves as having any control over their own health this did not mean that they were not interested in their health. All of them, for example, were acutely concerned with the prospect of progressing to ARC and AIDS even if they did not see themselves as having much control over this process:

> Sally talked about how she felt she did not know very much about AIDS/HIV. 'I'd like to know more. When I was up at the hospital I got a T4 cell count of 783 and I came back here and told ma drug counsellor who was over the moon so that was really good but I would like to know more, not to become obsessed or anything but just to know how long I had. I think though that by the time I get AIDS there'll be a cure'.

(Residential detoxification unit)

There is considerable scope for involving HIV positive drug injectors in health maintenance and health improvement initiatives have been employed among other groups of HIV infected individuals. These include relaxation therapies, massage, dietary changes and group therapy. An individual's continued drug use should never be seen as sufficient reason not involve drug injectors in locally existent or envisaged health initiatives.

Policy and service implications

We would draw attention to five areas for which we feel our work in this area has particular relevance.

First, the level of fear with which most drug injectors regarded AIDS and HIV should be noted. Whilst it obviously makes good sense to inform new drug injectors of the risks of HIV, there is also the danger of creating an atmosphere of such fear that individuals begin to avoid any information to do with the subject. There are signs that this is beginning to happen. It is worth remembering, too, that any media campaigns aiming to shock drug injectors into changing their behaviour are also going to be seen by those who are already having to cope with having an HIV positive diagnosis. It is clear from our work that many of these people are already extremely pessimistic as to what the future might hold. Any 'shock horror' approach then might lead to an increase in suicidal behaviour.

Second, as we noted earlier, many of the drug injectors we contacted had been tested because of other people's concern that they were injecting drug users. This should not happen and people should certainly not be informed of their results without adequate pre- and post-test counselling. Although it is worth remembering that very little is known about the effectiveness of counselling in this area.

Third, seropositive drug injectors should receive positive help with informing people about their HIV diagnosis and coping with requests to share their injecting equipment. It should *not* be assumed that provision of an HIV positive diagnosis will lead to a cessation in drug injecting. On some occasions this will happen, but on many occasions it will not. If individuals continue to inject drugs they will continue to be asked to pass on their injecting equipment to others. This being the case, seropositive drug injectors need to feel able to turn down such requests without feeling that they are thereby revealing their HIV positive status.

Fourth, many of the seropositive drug injectors saw little chance of their forming any long-term relationships with other people. There is no reason why this should be the case. Those involved in the care of HIV positive drug injectors should try to foster relationships between HIV positive individuals and others. This is unlikely to be an easy task and yet individuals should not feel that the diagnosis of being positive is equivalent to a social death. It is worth noting that a recent survey in the United States found a positive association between knowing someone who was HIV positive and tolerance of people with the virus (Gerbert *et al.* 1991). In the light of such a finding there should be a concerted attempt to prevent the marginalization of people with HIV infection.

Fifth, there is a good case for involving drug injectors in their own therapy. In part, this will entail providing them with more information on their own condition. It will also require fostering a belief amongst seropositive drug injectors that their health is something over which they can have some influence. However, one must take the references to suicidal behaviour very seriously. Ultimately HIV positive drug injectors need to be encouraged in the feeling that they can be HIV positive and still have much to live for.

We would like to end this chapter on a personal note. In many media reports drug injectors are portrayed as a dangerous group threatening others. Our lasting memory of the seropositive drug injectors we interviewed could hardly be more different. That image is of young people isolated, with little in the way of financial resources, having to cope with the reality of illness and death at a time when their lives ought to have been opening up before them.

Chapter 7

Conclusion

In each of the main chapters in this book we have outlined what we see as the main implications of our work for policy makers and service providers in the field of drug use and HIV. In this concluding chapter our purpose is not to reiterate what has gone before. Rather, we want to make a number of general points arising out of this work which have a bearing on efforts to change drug injectors' risk behaviour patterns. We will look then more critically at some of the social policy implications of our recommendations in relation to needle and syringe provision, heterosexual transmission of HIV and prostitution. In a final section we will look to what the future might hold as regards drug injectors and HIV.

First and foremost, it is important to stress how 'normal' the drug injectors were in their attitudes and behaviour. This is contrary to commonly held perceptions of drug injectors as individuals who are especially chaotic, and subject to unique and deviant motivations. In their fears about AIDS and HIV, in their difficulties with condom use, in their awkwardness over the whole issue of negotiating sex, in their hopes and expectations of family life, and in the way they sought to manage the attendant obligations of friendships, the drug injectors we contacted were indistinguishable from people in general.

Second, it is clear that knowledge of AIDS and HIV was widespread. However, it was also apparent that knowledge itself was not enough to change behaviour. This news is hardly a revelation since the field of health education is replete with examples where knowledge of the risks involved has not been sufficient to change behaviour, heart disease and diet, lung cancer and smoking being just two examples (Leviton 1989). It should not be assumed that simply informing people of the risks of sharing syringes and unprotected sex will in itself lead to a decrease in these risk behaviour patterns.

Third, it is clear from our study that the single most important factor complicating the relationship between knowledge and behaviour is that these are social behaviour patterns, embedded within social contexts. Situational and interpersonal factors are highly likely to exert strong influences which cut across straightforward injunctions to effect behaviour change. In Chapter 3, for example, we showed how the request to share injecting equipment could be influenced, among other things, by such factors as the local culture of sharing prevailing within an area, the nature of the relationship between injectors, obligations of friendship, and reciprocity between injectors and peer intimidation. The point is that each of these factors can exert an influence on behaviour over and above an individual's knowledge of the risks involved. A similar case can be made in relation to condom use. For instance, a woman might know and understand the risks of unprotected sex; nevertheless, the social stigma that often attaches to carrying condoms or the difficulties of introducing the topic of condom use within a long-term relationship, can mean, as we saw in Chapter 4, that condoms are not used and sexual risks are taken.

It is also important to stress, however, that difficult as it is to change behaviour this is not an impossible task given sufficient individual motivation or a supportive local culture. In Chapter 3 on sharing, for example, we saw how a few highly motivated individuals were going to quite extraordinary lengths to avoid sharing injecting equipment. Similarly, in Chapter 5 we saw how condom use was ubquitous amongst the female prostitutes in their contacts with clients. Amongst the female prostitutes a shared occupational culture supporting the use of condoms whilst working was no doubt influential in contributing to their widespread use. It was equally true, however, that in their private relationships, where that occupational culture would be that much less salient, condoms were only rarely used.

What then are the implications following on from these general points in relation to attempts to change drug injectors' risk behaviour? First, we would say that there is no longer a great need, at least within the United Kingdom, for national media campaigns stressing the HIV-associated risks of drug injectors making shared use of needles and syringes. Knowledge in this area, as we have already pointed out, seems very widespread. What is needed instead are a range of locally based interventions aimed at reducing needle and syringe sharing and also promoting wider use of condoms. In relation to needle and syringe sharing it is clearly important to provide drug injectors with easier access to sterile injecting equipment. However, simply providing the means for avoiding sharing will not eradicate the shared use of injecting equipment for the simple reason that sharing is embedded not only within the culture of drug injectors, but also that of the wider culture. This being the case there is some merit in trying to utilize aspects of the drug injectors' own culture to change behaviour. Work of this kind has been carried out with some degree of success in New York City (Friedman *et al.* 1990b). In Chapter 3 we commented on the possible value of social skills training with drug injectors. By using such an approach one could organize groups of injectors to look at the situations in which sharing injecting equipment often occurs and to role play different ways of declining requests to share without compromising the relationships between injectors.

A similar case could be made with regard to encouraging more widespread use of condoms. We would endorse approaches to make condoms more readily available to young people, whether at low cost or no cost. However, in itself this is unlikely to lead to major increases in the use of condoms unless supplemented by efforts to foster a more open attitude to the whole issue of sex in general. It is important to encourage people to look critically at their own attitudes towards sex and, furthermore, for some serious work to be done to try to remove or play down some of the taboo trappings surrounding the subject of sex. Whilst these remain so firmly in place it is difficult to see how such important issues as the negotiation of the sexual encounter can be explicitly acknowledged. To reach the point where men and women alike are able to be assertive in their sexual relationships does seem to require as a first step, the ability to acknowledge and discuss the issue. Such discussions need to become an integral part of sex education in schools. In particular, much may be gained by looking at the processes leading up to the sexual encounter. Explicit treatment of what is usually left implicit would provide a concrete means of exploring the various different ways in which to raise the topic of condoms and safer sex in general.

Needle and syringe provision

One of the most controversial aspects of attempts to change drug injectors' behaviour in relation to sharing has been the question of whether or not drug injectors should be provided with easier access to sterile injecting equipment. For many people there is little point in repeatedly exhorting drug injectors to stop sharing injecting equipment unless one is also going to provide them with the means to avoid sharing – one of those means being the provision of sterile injecting equipment. For some others, however, providing sterile injecting equipment is seen as equivalent to actively encouraging an illegal activity.

Representatives of these two divergent positions often appear to hold contrasting images of the typical drug injector. On the one hand drug injectors are characterized as individuals who are trying to do what they can in difficult circumstances to avoid infection. On the other hand, they are portrayed as deviant individuals with little or no regard for their own health or the health of others. As we have tried to show in this book neither of these stereotypes are wholly accurate; drug injectors are as varied as any other group of people.

Within the United Kingdom the fear that injecting drug users might spread HIV infection to the wider non-drug injecting population has led to the setting up of syringe exchange programmes in many cities. Needle and syringe provision has, however, been seen as something which ought to be under the control of medically trained staff. Whether this is appropriate remains an open question. We know from a wide range of studies, for example, that individuals often begin injecting in their mid-teens, usually with injecting equipment belonging to somebody else. To reduce sharing at the very earliest stages in the career of a drug injector neccessitates that needles and syringes be much more accessible to young people than is presently the case within the United Kingdom. However, to suggest that injecting equipment ought to be available in supermarkets and other settings frequented by young people will be an anathema to many. Nevertheless, so long as needle and syringe provision remains embedded within medical type establishments then its impact on the lives of young people will remain less than it could be.

Increasing access to injecting equipment is only one of the factors likely to contribute to a reduction in the spread of HIV amongst injecting drug users. In addition, there is a strong case for providing drug injectors with the means to sterilize injecting equipment. A number of North American cities have had considerable success with providing drug injectors with small bottles of bleach. Similar interventions could be utilized within those settings in which it would clearly be inappropriate to provide injecting equipment (for example, prisons and residential drug detoxification units). We ought not to ignore the sharing that is undoubtedly occurring within both of those settings.

Heterosexual transmission of HIV

Although the perception of 'risk groups' as distinct from 'risk practices' has been widely criticized, nevertheless the image of drug injectors as a homogeneous and somewhat self-enclosed group persists in the minds of many people. As we showed in Chapter 4, very many of the male drug injectors we contacted had non-injecting sexual partners. Similarly, despite a belief amongst many non-injectors that they would be able to recognize and avoid sexual contact with an injecting drug user, the visual cues being used were inevitably extremely crude. There can be little doubt that the heterosexual spread of HIV infection from injecting drug users to both men and women not injecting drugs is occurring and will continue to do so in the future.

The finding of low levels of condom use amongst injecting drug users is depressing. At the risk of being repetitive it is worth stressing again that in their attitudes to condoms drug injectors are no different to people generally. There are, it seems, very real difficulties in introducing condoms within the context of both short-term sexual encounters and long-term sexual relationships. Encouraging the much wider use of condoms undoubtedly requires a major shift in attitudes towards sex generally. In addition, a concerted attempt on the part of health educationalists and others should be made to stress the risks not only of *contracting* HIV infection, but also of *spreading* infection. Those drug injectors who are sexually involved with non-injecting partners need to be made aware of the potential risks they pose to their partners. Ultimately, injecting drug users (as amongst others) should be encouraged in the perception that in addition to being responsible for their own health they also bear some responsibility for the health of their partners.

Prostitution

There is a tendency in popular news reporting to represent prostitutes as a reservoir of infection threatening others. That perception is greater for female prostitutes than male prostitutes, though for no better reason than that our ignorance of male prostitutes is so great that even such prejudicial attitudes have not really had the scope to develop.

Whilst it is true that prostitutes sell sex, it is equally true that it is males who, in the main, buy sex. Moreover, one does not have to spend very much time in an area where sex is being sold to recognize that the range of individuals buying sex is as broad as the range of males in society itself. Nevertheless, the perception remains of those who sell sex as a deviant group involved in a stigmatized and illegal activity, set apart from those who buy sex. This sets the context for much of our thinking about prostitution. Such attitudes, for example, can make it extremely difficult for female and male prostitutes to make full use of existing health services without feeling that they will incur the disapprobation of staff. It makes little difference if such disapprobation is real or felt, the consequences of limited contact with official agencies remain the same. The illegality of prostitution also creates the ridiculous situation in which outreach workers can provide male and female prostitutes with condoms and sterile injecting equipment only to see these items used in legal proceedings against prostitutes. It is easy to blame the police for arresting prostitutes and to criticize the courts for imposing fines on them. Both the police and the courts, however, are carrying out the laws of the land. It is those laws which enshrine our prejudicial attitudes towards those who sell sex. It will only be with a change in the law and, more importantly, our attitudes that the situation for female and male prostitutes will significantly alter.

Increasing the legal control of prostitutes leads ultimately in only one direction which is to the adoption of increasingly covert styles of working. Prostitution is not removed by such measures, but simply made less visible. One of the by-products of such increasingly covert styles of working is likely to be that the scope for negotiating safer sex with clients is also reduced. Instead of being able to negotiate safer sex with clients at the kerbside, negotiations may need to take place within the client's car. Having once entered the car a woman may find herself in a much weaker position to insist upon such matters as the use of condoms.

Rather than further stigmatizing prostitutes and making them subject to increasing legal constraints, services should be developed which are specifically targeted at prostitutes and which adopt a user-friendly style of working. Prostitutes differ not only by gender, but also by whether or not they are injecting drug users; services may need to reflect such differences. In our own work there were many occasions when non-drug injecting prostitutes commented on their reluctance to attend a drop-in clinic which is largely used by drug injecting women.

Services directed at female and male prostitutes should be located at street level where prostitutes work and at the times of day they work. In addition, there is probably a need to combine any drop-in centres for prostitutes with outreach work for those men and women who are reluctant to attend any kind of official or semi-official setting

Finally, there needs to be an explicit recognition that those who sell sex comprise only one half of the equation. From our work it is clear that the pressure for unprotected sex arises from clients, some of whom are offering additional money for such services. In light of this it is important to target clients in outreach programmes. The difficulties associated with this are likely to be considerable. However, many clients walk around red-light areas, and are, therefore, open to being approached by outreach workers and provided with condoms. In our most recent work in Glasgow we have had some success in approaching clients in this way.

Changing fortunes: the future for injectors

At the time of writing this book one of the most optimistic recent reports has been to show the value of low dosages of the drug AZT in delaying the onset of symptoms in individuals with asymptomatic HIV infection. By using the drug in low dosages it now appears that the major side-effects of its use can be avoided making it possible to use the drug with a wider range of patients. This development is already having a major impact on the treatment of HIV infection and on the issue of HIV testing. Whereas previously there was little that could be offered to an individual testing HIV positive this is no longer the case. However, AZT remains an expensive drug (at the time of writing approximately £100 per 100 tablets). Whether the drug will be made equally available to all individuals infected with HIV remains to be seen. It may be that financial constraints within different health care systems will result in clinicians targeting the drug for certain patient groups in preference to others.

One of the most heated arguments currently taking place within the field of drug use and HIV infection concerns the role of substitute prescribing. Basically, this has to do with whether or not HIV positive drug injectors should be offered oral or injectable methadone and ultimately whether they should be offered heroin. In some ways it is an indictment of service providers and others that there have not been equivalent calls for the wider use of AZT with injecting drug users. At the Seventh International Conference on AIDS (Florence, 1991) there was some debate as to whether or not the continued use of drugs such as methadone and heroin by individuals with damaged immune systems could lead to more rapid disease progression. If this does prove to be the case, deciding whether to provide drug injectors with methadone or heroin will take on a quite different character.

Whilst the story in relation to AZT seems relatively positive, the continuation of risk behaviour amongst injecting drug users described in this study as (well as in numerous others) is rather less so. At present it is simply not known what level of risk behaviour within a population is sufficient to generate a local epidemic of HIV infection. It may be that even those changes in risk behaviour which have been variously documented among injectors will be insufficient to stop the spread of HIV infection amongst injecting drug users. On a global scale it seems highly likely that HIV will continue to spread amongst injecting drug users. National governments ought not to feel impotent in the face of the challenge represented by AIDS and HIV. It is probable, for example, that the limited spread of HIV among injecting drug users in Australia is, in a large part, due to the speed and vigour with which harm reduction policies were instituted and carried out there (Wodak 1990).

The key to stopping the spread of AIDS and HIV among injecting drug users, however, rests not with methadone, AZT, heroin, sterile injecting equipment or condoms, but with addressing the very basis of injecting drug use in the first place. It makes little sense to spend endless hours attempting to prove or disprove whether unemployment and poverty cause drug use. The simple fact remains that such behaviour flourishes where young people see nothing positive in their own lives or in the lives of others around them. AIDS and HIV present many complex challenges in almost every area of human life. Yet, difficult as those challenges are, they can seem minute compared to the societal changes necessary to induce a sense of value and positive future in young peoples' lives. In this area, as in others, the discourse of risk behaviour, treatments and vaccines glosses over more fundamental and political concerns which remain largely unaddressed. However, until they are confronted and until major economic changes are brought about (which at minimum address unemployment), the unpalatable truth remains that young people will continue to inject as a means of providing excitement and purpose to their lives, and continue also to pay the cost with their diminished health and premature death.

Glossary of local terms

A doin': A beating up
A heavy: An aggressive and influential individual
Back close: Rear stairwell in a tenement
Barrel: Syringe
Batterin': A beating up
Bogging: Dirty
Chokin': Desperate for drug injection
Deid: Dead, deceased
Durex: Condom
Eggs: Temazepam
Fag: Cigarette
Full of it: Experiencing the effects of recent drug use
Gouch: Drug induced stupor
Greetin': Crying
Hep: Hepatitis B
Hitting: Injecting
Jellies: Temazepam
Junk: Heroin
Kidologists: Conmen, people who attempt to fool others
Kit: Heroin
Manky: Dirty
Midden: Dirty, often used to refer to a person
Poke: Paper bag
Polis: Police
Rattlin': Experiencing symptoms of drug withdrawal
Scheme: Local Authority housing estate
Score deal: £20 bag of heroin
Shot through: Broken or not functioning
Smack: Heroin
Spike: Needle

Squared up: Able to function at a minimum level
Stairwell: Stairs in a tenement block
Stank: Drain/sewer
Steamin': Drunk
Strung out: Drug withdrawal
Sulph: Amphetamine sulphate
Tems: Temgesic
Tools: Injecting equipment
Wean: Child
Works: Injecting equipment

References

Abrams, D., Abraham, C., Spears, R. and Marks, D. (1990). 'AIDS invulnerability: relationships, sexual behaviour and attitudes among 16–19 year olds', in P. Aggleton, P. Davies and G. Hart (eds) *AIDS: Individual, Cultural and Policy Dimensions*. Brighton, Falmer Press.

Andiman, W., Simpson, B., Olsen, B. *et al.* (1990). 'Rate of transmission of Human Immunodeficiency Virus Type 1 infection from mother to child and short-term outcome of neonatal infection', *American Journal of Diseases of Children*, 144, 758–66.

Answer (AIDS News Supplement, CDS Weekly Report) (1990a). 'WHO issues new estimates on global AIDS situation' (CDS 90/50).

Answer (AIDS News Supplement, CDS Weekly Report) (1990b). 'Human Immunodeficiency Virus (HIV) infection', Scotland Quarterly Report to 30 September 1990 (CDS 90/41).

Arras, J. (1990). 'AIDS and reproductive decisions: having children in fear and trembling', *Millbank Quarterly*, 68, 353–82.

Barnard, M.A. (1991). 'Working in the dark: researching female prostitution', in H. Roberts (ed.) *Women's Health Matters*. London, Routledge.

Barnard, M.A. and McKeganey, N.P. (1990). 'Adolescents, sex and injecting drug use: risks for HIV infection', *AIDS Care*, 2, 103–16.

Battjes, R., Pickens, R. and Amsel, Z. (1989). 'Introduction of HIV infection among intravenous drug abusers in low prevalence areas', *Journal of the Acquired Immune Deficiency Syndrome*, 2, 533–9.

Baxter, L. A. and Wilmot, W.W. (1985). 'Taboo topics in close relationships', *Journal of Social and Personal Relationships*, 2, 253–69.

Bayer, R. (1991). 'AIDS and the future of reproductive freedom', in D. Nelkin, D. Willis, S. Parris (eds) *A Disease of Society: Cultural and Institutional Responses to AIDS*. Cambridge, Cambridge University Press.

Blanche, S.C., Rouzioux, M., Moscato, L. *et al.* (1989). 'A prospective study of infants born to women seropositive for Human Immunodeficiency Virus Type 1', *New England Journal of Medicine*, 320, 1643–8.

Bloor, M.J., Rahman, M.Z., McKeganey, N.P. *et al.* (1989). 'Needle sharing in residential drug treatment units' (letter), *British Journal of Addiction*, 84, 1547–9.

Bloor, M. J., Barnard, M., Finlay, A. and McKeganey, N. (1991a). 'HIV related risk practices among Glasgow male prostitutes', paper presented to BSA Annual Conference, Manchester.

Bloor, M.J., Goldberg, D. and Emslie, J. (1991b). 'Ethnostatistics and the AIDS epidemic', *British Journal of Sociology*, 42, 130–8.

Bloor, M.J., McKeganey, N.P. and Barnard, M.A. (1990). 'An ethnographic study of male prostitution and risks of HIV spread in Glasgow: a report of a pilot study', *AIDS Care*, 2, 17–24.

Broadhead, R.S. and Fox, K.J. (1990). 'Takin' it to the streets: AIDS outreach as ethnography', *Journal of Contemporary Ethnography*, 19, 332–48.

Brooks-Gunn, J. and Furstenberg, J.R.F. (1990). 'Coming of age in the era of AIDS: puberty, sexuality and contraception', *Millbank Quarterly*, 68, 59–84.

Brunet, J.B., Des Jarlais, D.C. and Koch, M.A. (1987). 'Report on the European Community Workshop on the epidemiology of HIV infections: spread among intravenous drug abusers and the heterosexual population', *AIDS*, 1, 59–61.

Callen, M. (1989). 'Living with AIDS and HIV', *AIDS Forum*, 3, 16–22.

Calsyn, D.A., Saxon, A.J., Freeman, G. and Whittaker, S. (1991). 'Needle-use practices among intravenous drug users in an area where needle purchase is legal', *AIDS*, 5, 187–93.

Chaisson, M.A., Stoneburner R.L., Lifson, A.R. *et al.* (1990). 'Risk factors for Human Immunodeficiency Virus Type 1 HIV-1 infection in patients at a sexually transmitted disease clinic in New York City', *American Journal of Epidemiology*, 131, 208–20.

Chaisson, R.E., Moss, A.R., Onishi, R. *et al.* (1987). 'Human Immunodeficiency Virus infection in heterosexual intravenous drug users in San Francisco', *American Journal of Public Health*, 77, 169–72.

Chin, J. (1990). 'Current and future dimensions of the HIV/AIDS pandemic in women and children', *The Lancet*, 336, 221–4.

Chin, J. and Mann, J.M. (1988). 'Global patterns and prevalence of AIDS and HIV infection', *AIDS*, 2 (Suppl. 1), S247–52.

Cohen, J., Hauer, L. and Wofsy, C. (1989). 'Women and IV drugs: parenteral and heterosexual transmission of Human Immunodeficiency Virus', *Journal of Drug Issues*, 19, 39–56.

Cohen, J.B. (1989). 'Overstating the risk of AIDS: scapegoating prostitutes', *Focus, A Guide to AIDS Research*, 4, 1–2.

Coleman, R.M. and Curtis, D. (1988). 'Distribution of risk behaviour for HIV infection amongst intravenous drug users', *British Journal of Addiction*, 83, 1331–4.

Cowan, F.M., Flegg, P.J. and Brettle, R.P. (1989). 'Heterosexually acquired HIV infection' (letter), *British Medical Journal*, 298, 891.

Coxon, A.P. and Carballo, M. (1989). Editorial Review, 'Research on AIDS: behavioural perspectives', *AIDS*, 3, 191–7.

Cruz, E. (1989). 'The other half I got to live', *The Body Positive*, May, 3, 13–14.

D'Costa, L.J., Plummer, F.A., Bowner, J. *et al.* (1985). 'Prostitutes are a major reservoir of transmitted diseases in Nairobi, Kenya', *Sexually Transmitted Diseases*, 12, 64–7.

Day, S. (1988). 'Prostitute women and AIDS: anthropology', *AIDS*, 2, 421–8.

Day, S., Ward, H. and Harris, J.R.W. (1988). 'Prostitute women and public health', *British Medical Journal*, 297, 1585.

Defoe, D. (1986) *A Journal of The Plague Years* (first published in 1772). London, Penguin Classics.

Des Jarlais, D.C. and Friedman, S.R. (1990). 'The epidemic of HIV infection among injecting drug users in New York City: the first decade and possible future directions', in J. Strang and G. Stimson (eds) *AIDS and Drug Misuse: The Challenge for Policy and Practice in the 1990's*. London, Routledge.

Des Jarlais, D.C., Friedman, S.R. and Stoneburner, R. (1988). 'HIV infection and intravenous drug use: critical issues in transmission dynamics, infection outcomes, and prevention', *Review of Infectious Diseases*, 10, 151–9.

Des Jarlais, D.C., Friedman, S.R. and Strug, D. (1986). 'AIDS and needle sharing within the IV-drug use subculture', in D.A. Feldman and T.M. Johnson (eds) *Social Dimensions of AIDS: Method and Theory*. New York, Praeger.

Des Jarlais, D.C. and Friedman, S.R. (1987). 'Editorial Review: HIV infection among intravenous drug users: epidemiology and risk reduction', *AIDS*, 1, 67–76.

Des Jarlais, D.C., Wish, E., Friedman, S.R. *et al.* (1987). 'Intravenous drug use and the heterosexual transmission of the Human Immunodeficiency Virus: current trends in New York City', *New York State Journal of Medicine*, May, 283–6.

Doerr, H.W., Enzenberger, R., Bolender, C. *et al.* (1990). 'Prevalence of HIV infection in prostitutes from Frankfurt, W.Germany', Poster at Sixth International Conference on AIDS, San Francisco, USA.

Donoghoe, M.C., Stimson, G.V. and Dolan, K.A. (1989). 'Sexual behaviour of injecting drug users and associated risks of HIV infection for non-injecting sexual partners', *AIDS Care*, 1, 51–8.

Douglas, M. (1966). *Purity and Danger: An Analysis of Concepts of Pollution and Taboo*. London, Routledge.

Dreuilhe, E. (1989). *Mortal Embrace – Living With AIDS*. London, Faber and Faber.

Dumont, L. (1970). *Homo Hierarchicus: the Caste System and its Implications*. London, Weidenfeld and Nicolson.

European Collaborative Study (1991). 'Children born to mothers with HIV-1 infection: natural history and risk of transmission', *Lancet*, 337, 253–9.

Feldman, H.W. and Biernacki, P. (1988). 'The ethnography of needle sharing among intravenous drug users and implications for public policies and intervention strategies', in R.J. Battjes and R.W. Pickens (eds) *Needle Sharing Among Intravenous Drug Abusers: National and International Perspectives*, NIDA Research Monograph 80. Rockville, MD.

Fields, A. and Walters, J.M. (1985). 'Hustling: supporting a heroin habit', in B. Hanson, G. Beschner, J.M. Walters and E. Bovelle (eds) *Life with Heroin, Voices from the Inner City*. Lexington, Mass. Lexington Books.

Follett E., McIntyre, A., O'Donnell, B. *et al.* (1986). 'HTLV-III antibody in drug abusers in the west of Scotland: The Edinburgh connection' (letter), *Lancet*, 14 February, 446–7.

Friedman, S.R., Des Jarlais, D.C., Neaigus, A. *et al.* (1989). 'AIDS and the new drug injector', *Nature*, 339, 333–4.

Friedman, S.R., Des Jarlais, D.C. and Sterk, C. (1990a). 'AIDS and the social relations of intravenous drug users', *Millbank Quarterly*, 86 (Suppl. 1), 85–110.

Friedman, S.R., Sterk, C., Sufian, M. *et al.* (1990b). 'Reaching out to injecting drug users', in J. Strang and G.V. Stimson (eds) *AIDS and Drug Misuse: The Challenge for Policy and Practice in the 1990's*. London, Routledge.

Frischer, M.J. (1991). 'Estimated prevalence of injecting drug use in Glasgow', *British Journal of Addiction*, in press.

Frischer, M., Bloor, M., Finlay, A. *et al.* (1991). 'A new method of estimating prevalence of injecting drug use in an urban population: results from a Scottish city', *International Journal of Epidemiology*, 20, 997–1000.

Gerbert, B., Sumser, J. and Maguire, B.T. (1991). 'The impact of who you know and where you live on opinions about AIDS and health care', *Social Science and Medicine*, 32, 677–81.

Gillman, C. and Feldman, H. (1991). 'When love can't protect: the sexual transmission of HIV', Paper presented to the Second International Conference on the Reduction of Drug Related Harm, Barcelona, Spain, 1991.

Godlee, F. (1990). 'Dutch example of teenage sexuality', *British Medical Journal*, 301, 551.

Goldberg, D.J., Green, S.J., Kingdom, J.C.P. and Christie, P.R. (1988a). 'HIV infection among female drug abusing prostitutes in Greater Glasgow', *ANSWER: Supplement to Communicable Diseases, Scotland, Weekly Report*, 22 (12).

Goldberg, D.J., Watson, H., Stuart, F. *et al.* (1988b). 'Pharmacy supply of needles and syringes', *IVth International Conference on AIDS*, June 1988, Stockholm (Abs 8521).

Golden, E., Fullilove, M., Fullilove, R. *et al.* (1990). 'The effects of gender and crack use on high risk behaviours', *VI International Conference on AIDS*, June, 1990, San Francisco (Abs 742).

Grund, J.P., Kaplan, C., Adriaans, N. and Blanken, P. (1991). 'Drug sharing and HIV transmission risks: the practice of frontloading in the Dutch injecting drug user population', *Journal of Psychoactive Drugs*, 23, 1.

Haw, S., Covell, R., Finlay, A. and Frischer, M. *et al*, (1991). 'A serial period prevalence study of HIV infection and HIV risk behaviour among a sample of injecting drug users', *V11 International Conference on AIDS*, Florence (MD4070).

Haw, S. (1985). *Drug Problems in Greater Glasgow: Report of the SCODA Fieldwork Survey in Greater Glasgow Health Board*. Glasgow, SCODA.

Hearst, N. and Hulley, S.B. (1988). 'Preventing the heterosexual spread of AIDS. Are we giving our patients the best advice?' *Journal of the American Medical Association*, 259, 2428–32.

Holland, J., Ramazanoglu, C., Scott, S. and Thomson, R. (1990a). '"Don't die of ignorance" – I nearly died of embarrassment: condoms in context', paper presented at *Fourth Conference on Social Aspects of AIDS*, April 1990, South Bank Polytechnic, London.

Holland, J., Ramazanoglu, C., Scott, S. *et al.* (1990b). 'Sex, gender and power: young women's sexuality in the shadow of AIDS', *Sociology of Health and Illness*, 12, 336–50.

Horowitz, R. (1981). 'Passion, submission and motherhood: the negotiation of identity by unmarried inner city Chicanas', *Sociological Quarterly*, 22, 241–52.

Howard, J. and Borges, P. (1970). 'Needle sharing in the Haight: some social and psychological functions', *Journal of Health and Social Behaviour*, 11, 220–30.

Jackson, S. (1982). *Childhood and Sexuality*. Oxford, Basil Blackwell.

James, A. (1986). 'Learning to belong: the boundaries of adolescence', in A. Cohen (ed.) *Symbolising Boundaries: Identity and Diversity in British Cultures*. Manchester, Manchester University Press.

James, J., Gosho, C. and Watson-Wohl, R. (1979). 'The relationship between female criminality and drug use', *International Journal of the Addictions*, 14, 215–29.

Joseph, S. (1989). Kenneth, D. Blackfan Lecture 'Paediatric AIDS in New York City: a perspective from the epicenter', Boston, June 7.

Kane, S. (1991). 'HIV, heroin and heterosexual relations', *Social Science and Medicine*, 32, 1037–50.

Kent, V., Davies, M., Deverell, K. and Gottesman, S. (1990). 'Social interaction routines involved in heterosexual encounters: prelude to first intercourse', paper presented at *Fourth Conference on Social Aspects of AIDS*, 7 April, South Bank Polytechnic, London.

Kinnell, H. (1989). 'Prostitutes, their clients and risks of HIV Infection in Birmingham', *Occasional Paper*, Department of Public Health Medicine, Birmingham.

Kitzinger, J. (1990). 'The face of AIDS', paper given at Medical Sociology Conference, Edinburgh, 14–16 September.

Klee, H. (1990). 'Some observations on the sexual behaviour of injecting drug users: implications for the spread of HIV infection', in P. Aggleton, P. Davies and G. Hart (eds) *AIDS: Individual, Cultural and Policy Dimensions*. Brighton, Falmer Press, 155–68.

Klee, H., Faugier, J., Hayes, C. *et al.* (1990). 'AIDS-related risk behaviour, polydrug use and temazepam', *British Journal of Addiction*, 85, 1125–32.

Kleinegris, M. (1991). 'Innovative AIDS prevention among drug using prostitutes', paper presented to Second International Conference on the Reduction of Drug Related Harm, Barcelona, Spain.

Lange, W.R., Snyder, F.R., Lozovsky, D. *et al.* (1987). 'HIV infection in Baltimore: antibody seroprevalence rates among parenteral drug abusing prostitutes', *Maryland Medical Journal*, 36, 757–61.

Lawrinson, S. (1991). 'Prostitutes and safe sexual practice', paper presented at BSA Annual Conference, Manchester.

Levine, L. C. and Neveloff Dubler, N. (1990). 'HIV and childbearing, uncertain risks and bitter realities: the reproductive choices of HIV infected women', *Millbank Quarterly*, 68, 321–51.

Leviton, L. (1989). 'Theoretical foundations of AIDS – prevention programs', in R.O. Valderserri (ed.) *Preventing AIDS: The Design of Effective Programs*. New Brunswick, Rutgers University Press.

Liebow, E. (1967). *Tally's Corner: A Study of Negro Street Corner Men*. Boston, USA, Little Brown Publishers.

Macdonald, G. and Smith, C. (1990). 'Complacency, risk perception and the problem of HIV education', *AIDS Care*, 2, 63–8.

Marmor, M., Des Jarlais, D.C., Cohen, H. *et al.* (1987). 'Risk factors for infection with Human Immunodeficiency Virus among intravenous drug abusers in New York City', *AIDS*, 1, 39–44.

McCann, K. and Wadsworth, E. (1991). 'The experience of having a positive HIV antibody test', *AIDS Care*, 3, 43–53.

McKeganey, N.P. (1990). 'Being positive: drug injectors experiences of HIV infection', *British Journal of Addiction*, 85, 1113–24.

McKeganey, N.P., Barnard, M.A., Bloor, M.J. and Leyland, A.C. (1990a). 'Injecting drug use and female streetworking prostitution in Glasgow', *AIDS*, 1, 1153–5.

McKeganey, N.P., Barnard, M.A. and Bloor, M.J. (1990b). 'A comparison of HIV related risk behaviour and risk reduction between female streetworking prostitutes and male rent boys in Glasgow', *Sociology of Health and Illness*, 12, 274–92.

McKeganey, N.P., Barnard, M.A. and Watson, H. (1989). 'HIV related risk behaviour among a non-clinic sample of injecting drug users', *British Journal of Addiction*, 84, 1481–90.

McMullen, R. (1988). *Living with HIV in Self and Others*. London, Gay Men Press.

Mitchell, J. (1988). 'Women, AIDS and public policy', *AIDS and Public Policy Journal*, 3, 50–2.

Mittag, H. (1991). 'AIDS prevention and sexual liberalisation in Great Britain', *Social Science and Medicine*, 32, 783–91.

(*Mortality and Morbidity Weekly Report MMWR, Centers for Disease Control, Atlanta, U.S.A.*) (1989). 'Current trends, update: heterosexual transmission of Acquired Immunodeficiency Syndrome and Human Immunodeficiency Virus infection – United States', 38 (24), 429–34.

MMWR (Morbidity and Mortality Weekly Report Centers for Disease Control) (1987). 'Epidemiologic notes and reports: antibody of human immunodeficiency virus in female prostitutes', 36 (11), 157–61.

Morgan Thomas, R., Plant, M.A., Plant, M.L. and Sales, D.I. (1989). 'Risk of AIDS among workers in the sex industry: some initial results from a Scottish Study', *British Medical Journal*, 299, 148–9.

Muga, R., Tor, J., Jacas, C. *et al.* (1990). 'Risk factors for HIV I infection in parenteral drug abusers', Sixth International Conference on AIDS, San Francisco (FC 643).

Mulleady, G. and Sherr, L. (1989). 'Lifestyle factors for drug users in relation to risks for HIV', *AIDS Care*, 1, 45–50.

Naik, T.N., Sarkar, S., Singh, H. *et al.* (1991). 'Intravenous drug users – a new high risk group for HIV infection in India', *AIDS*, 5, 117–18.

Nicolosi, A. (1990). 'Different susceptibility of woman and man to heterosexual transmission of HIV', *VI International Conference on AIDS*, San Francisco (THC 585).

Norman, S., Studd, J. and Johnson, A. (1990). 'HIV infection in women', *British Medical Journal*, 301, 1231–32.

Novick, L.F., Berns, D. and Stricof, R. (1989). 'HIV seroprevalence in new-borns in New York State', *Journal of the American Medical Association*, 261, 1745–50.

Nutbeam, D. (1989). 'Public knowledge and attitudes to AIDS', *Journal of Public Health*, 103, 205–211.

Padian, N. (1987). 'Heterosexual transmission of Acquired Immunodeficiency Syndrome: International perspectives and national projections', *Review of Infectious Diseases*, 9, 947–59.

Padian, N.S. (1988). 'Prostitute women and AIDS: epidemiology', *AIDS*, 6, 413–19.

Parker, H., Bakx, K. and Newcombe, R. (1988). *Living with Heroin*. Milton Keynes, Open University Press.

Patrick, J. (1973). *A Glasgow Gang Observed*. London, Eyre Methuen.

Pearson, G. (1987). *The New Heroin Users*. London, Blackwell.

Peckham, C.S. and Newell, M.L. (1990). 'HIV-1 infection in mothers and babies' (Editorial), *AIDS Care*, 2, 205–11.

Perlmutter Bowen, S. and Michel-Johnson, P. (1989). 'The crisis of communicating in relationships: confronting the threat of AIDS', *AIDS and Public Policy Journal*, 4, 10–19.

Piot, P., Plummer, F.A., D'Costa, L.J. *et al.* (1987). 'Retrospective seroepidemiology of AIDS virus infection in Nairobi populations', *Journal of Infectious Diseases*, 155, 1108–12.

Pizzo, P.A. (1989). 'Emerging concepts of the treatment of HIV infection in children', *Journal of the American Medical Association*, 262,1989–92.

Pollack, L., Ekstrand, M.L., Stall, R. and Coates, T.J. (1990). 'Current reasons for having unsafe sex among gay men in San Francisco: The AIDS Behavioural Research Project', Poster at Sixth International Conference on AIDS, San Francisco, U.S.A.

Pollack, S. (1985). 'Sex and the contraceptive act', in H. Homans (ed.) *The Sexual Politics of Reproduction*. London, Gower Press.

Power, R. (1988). 'The influence of AIDS upon patterns of intravenous use – syringe and needle sharing among illicit drug users in Britain', in R.J. Battjes and R.W. Pickens (eds) *Needle Sharing Among Intravenous Drug Abusers: National and International Perspectives*, NIDA Research Monograph 80.

Public Health Laboratory Service Collaborative Study Group (1989). 'HIV infection in patients attending clinics for sexually transmitted diseases in England and Wales', *British Medical Journal*, 298, 415–18.

Rezza, G., Titti, F., Tempesta, E. *et al.* (1989). 'Needle sharing and other behaviours related to HIV spread among intravenous drug users' (letter), *AIDS*, 3, 247–8.

Richardson, D. (1990). 'AIDS education and women: sexual and reproductive issues', in P. Aggleton, P. Davies and G. Hart (eds) *AIDS: Individual, Cultural and Policy Dimensions*. Brighton, Falmer Press.

Robertson, J.R., Bucknall, A.B.V., Welsby, P. *et al.* (1986). 'Epidemic of AIDS related virus (HTLV-III/LAV): infection among intravenous drug abusers', *British Medical Journal*, 292, 527–9.

Robertson, J.R. and Skidmore, C. (1989). 'Heterosexually acquired HIV infection' (letter), *British Medical Journal*, 298, 891.

Robertson, J.R., Skidmore, C.A. and Roberts, J.J.K. (1988). 'HIV infection in intravenous drug users: a follow-up study indicating changes in risk-taking behaviour', *British Journal of Addiction*, 83, 387–91.

Robertson, J.R. (1990). 'The Edinburgh Epidemic: a case study', in J. Strang and G. Stimson (eds) *AIDS and Drug Misuse: The Challenge for Policy and Practice in the 1990's*. London, Routledge.

Robinson, T. (1989). 'London's homosexual male prostitutes: power, peer groups and HIV', Working Paper 12, *Project Sigma*, London, South Bank Polytechnic.

Rosenbaum, M. (1981). 'Sex roles among deviants: the woman addict', *International Journal of the Addictions*, 16, 859–77.

Rosenberg, M.J. and Weiner, N. (1988). 'Prostitutes and AIDS: a Health Department priority?', *American Journal of Public Health*, 78, 418–23.

Sakol, M.S., Stark, C. and Sykes, R. (1989). 'Buprenorphine and temazepam abuse by drug takers in Glasgow – an increase', *British Journal of Addiction*, 84, 439–41.

Sandstrom, K.L. (1990). 'Confronting deadly disease: the drama of identity construction among gay men with AIDS', *Journal of Contemporary Ethnography*, 19, 271–94.

Sato, P., Chin, J. and Mann, J. (1989). 'Review of AIDS and HIV infection: global epidemiology and statistics', *AIDS*, 3 (Suppl. 1), S301–7.

Schutz, A. (1970). *Reflections on the Problem of Relevance*. New Haven and London, Yale University Press.

Scott, S. (1987). 'Sex and danger: feminism and AIDS', *Trouble and Strife*, 11, 13–18.

Selwyn, P., Carter, R., Schoenbaum, E. *et al.* (1990). 'Knowledge of HIV antibody status and decisions to continue or terminate pregnancy among intravenous drug users', *Journal of the American Medical Association*, 261, 3567–71.

Shapiro, C.N., Lloyd Schultz, S., Lee, N. and Dondero, T. (1989). 'Review of Human Immunodeficiency Virus infection in women in the United States', *Journal of Obstetrics and Gynaecology*, 74, 800–8.

Shedlin, M. (1990). 'An ethnographic approach to understanding HIV high risk behaviour: prostitution and drug abuse', in C.J. Leukefeld, R.J. Battjes and Z. Amsel (eds) *AIDS and Intravenous Drug Use: Community Interventions and Prevention*. New York, Hemisphere Publishing Corporation, pp. 134–49.

Siegel, K. and Krauss, B.J. (1991). 'Living with infection: adaptive tasks of seropositive gay men', *Journal of Health and Social Behaviour*, 32, 17–32.

Skidmore, C.A., Robertson, J.R. and Savage, G. (1990). 'Mortality and increasing drug use in Edinburgh: implications for the HIV epidemic', *Scottish Medical Journal*, 35, 100–2.

Sonenstein, F.L., Pleck, J.H. and Leighton, C.K. (1989). 'Sexual activity, condom use and AIDS awareness among adolescent males', *Family Planning Perspectives*, 21, 152–8.

Stein, Z.A. (1990). 'HIV prevention: the need for methods women can use', *American Journal of Public Health*, 80, 460–2.

Stimson, G.V. (1987). 'The war on heroin: British policy and the international trade in illicit drugs', in N. Dorn and N. South (eds) *A Land fit for Heroin? Drug Policies, Prevention and Practice*. London, Macmillan.

Stimson, G.V., Donoghoe, M., Aldritt, L. and Dolan, K. (1988). 'HIV transmission risk behaviour of clients attending syringe exchange schemes in England and Scotland', *British Journal of Addiction*, 53, 1449–55.

Stoneburner, R., Chaisson, M.A., Weifuse, I. and Thomas, P.A. (1990). 'The epidemic of AIDS and HIV–1 infection among heterosexuals in New York City', *AIDS*, 4, 99–106.

Tempesta E. and Giannantonio, M. (1988). 'Sharing needles and the spread of HIV in Italy's addict population', in R. Battjes and W. Pickens (eds) *Needle Sharing Among Intravenous Drug Abusers: National and International Perspectives*, Research Monograph series 80. Washington, National Institute on Drug Abuse.

Tempesta E. and Giannantonio, M. (1990). 'The Italian epidemic: a case study', in J. Strang and G. Stimson (eds) *AIDS and Drug Misuse: The Challenge for Policy and Practice in the 1990's*. London, Routledge.

Thomas, P., O'Donnell, R. *et al.* (1988). 'HIV infection in heterosexual female intravenous drug users in New York City', *New England Journal of Medicine,* 319, 374.

Tirelli, U., Rezza, G., Guiliani, M. *et al.* (1989). 'HIV seroprevalence among 304 female prostitutes from four Italian towns', *AIDS*, 3, 547–548.

van den Hoek, J.A.R., van Haastrecht, H.J.A. and Coutinho, R.A. (1990). 'Behavioural change in addicted prostitute women', Sixth International Conference on AIDS, San Francisco, (Abs. 3042).

van den Hoek, J.A.R., Coutinho, R.A., van Haastrecht, H.J.A., *et al.* (1988). 'Prevalence and risk factors of HIV infections among drug users and drug using prostitutes in Amsterdam', *AIDS*, 1, 55–60.

van den Hoek, J.A.R., van Haastrecht, H.J.A., Scheeringa-Troost, B., *et al.* (1989). 'HIV infection and STD in drug-addicted prostitutes in Amsterdam: potential for heterosexual HIV transmission', *Journal of Genitourinary Medicine*, 65, 146–50.

Vanichseni, S., Sakuntanaga, P. *et al.* (1990). 'Results of three seroprevalence surveys for HIV in IVDU in Bangkok', Sixth International Conference on AIDS, San Francisco (FC105).

Waldorf, D. and Murphy, S. (1990). 'IV drug use and syringe sharing practices of call men and hustlers', in M. Plant (ed.) *AIDS, Drugs and Prostitution*. London, Routledge.

Ward, H., Day, S., Donegan, C. and Harris, J.R.W. (1990). 'HIV risk behaviour and STD incidence in London prostitutes', Sixth International Conference on AIDS, San Francisco (FC 738).

Weinstein, S.A. and Goebel, G. (1979). 'The relationship between contraceptive sex role stereotyping and attitudes towards male contraception among males', *Journal of Sex Research*, 15, 235–42.

Weissman, G., Sowder, B. and Young, P. (1990). 'The relationship between crack cocaine use and other risk factors among women in a National AIDS Prevention Program – U.S., Puerto Rico and Mexico' Sixth International Conference on AIDS, San Francisco (SD 124).

Wellings, K. (1988). 'Other indicators of response to the AIDS Public Education Campaign', in *Health Education Authority Report*, September. London, HMSO.

Wight, O. (1990). 'The impact of HIV/AIDS on young people's heterosexual behavior: a literature Review', MRC Medical Sociology Unit working paper, No. 20.

Wodak, A. (1990). 'AIDS and injecting drug use in Australia: a case study in policy development and implementation', in J. Strang and G.V. Stimson (eds) *AIDS and Drug Misuse. The Challenge for Policy and Practice in the 1990's*. London, Routledge.

Name index

Subject index